Dr. Earl Mindell's

What You Should
Know About
22 Ways
to a
Healthier Heart

Dr. Earl Mindell's

What You Should Know About 22 Ways to a Healthier Heart

Earl L. Mindell, R.Ph., Ph.D.

with Virginia L. Hopkins

Keats Publishing, Inc.   New Canaan, Connecticut

DR. EARL MINDELL'S WHAT YOU SHOULD KNOW ABOUT 22 WAYS TO A HEALTHIER HEART

Copyright © 1996 by Earl L. Mindell, R.Ph., Ph.D.

All Rights Reserved

No part of this book may be reproduced in any form without the written consent of the publisher.

Library of Congress Cataloging-in-Publication Data
Mindell, Earl.
    [What you should know about 22 ways to a healthier heart]
    Dr. Earl Mindell's What you should know about 22 ways to a healthier heart : how to protect yourself naturally from America's number one killer / by Dr. Earl Mindell, with Virginia L. Hopkins.
        p. cm.
    Includes bibliographical references and index.
ISBN 0-87983-752-7
    1. Heart—Diseases—Prevention. I. Hopkins, Virginia. II. Title.
RC682.M56 1996
616.1'205—dc20   95-47348
                                                      CIP

Printed in the United States of America

Keats Publishing, Inc.
27 Pine Street (Box 876)
New Canaan, Connecticut 06840-0876

99 98 97 96   6 5 4 3 2 1

Contents

INTRODUCTION

Preventing Heart Disease Is Easier Than You Think

We all know somone who has died from a heart attack. Heart disease is by far the number one killer of Americans, and yet it is one of the simplest diseases to prevent. Even if your parents and grandparents had heart disease, you can still prevent it in yourself by following some simple guidelines, which I will give you in this book.

If heart disease kills more people every year than anything else, why aren't these simple cures being shouted from the rooftops? Why isn't it the biggest topic of discussion on all the talk shows? First of all, it's too simple, too inexpensive, and not nearly dramatic enough for a talk show. At the same time these simple cures are the hardest thing to do for many people, because they involve a change in lifestyle and daily habits.

The typical physician believes his or her patients won't make lifestyle changes, and doesn't even recommend them, even though it is well established that they work better than any drug ever has. In truth, your physician doesn't have the time to help you make lifestyle changes—writing out a prescription is quicker and easier. An expensive drug is prescribed that suppresses the symptoms of heart disease, such as high blood pressure or high cholesterol, and causes a whole range of unpleasant side effects. Pretty soon you're taking other drugs to treat the side effects of the first drugs, and you're on what I call the drug treadmill.

I'm going to tell you how to change your lifestyle and how to get off the drug treadmill. It's important not to go off drugs suddenly. I'd like you to work with your physician.

Many physicians will resist taking their patients off these drugs, because they make the numbers (blood pressure and cholesterol levels) look good. But suppressing these symptoms does not make the heart disease go away! I want you to work on the *causes* of heart disease. If you take the initiative to make positive changes in your diet, get some exercise, lose some weight and take some supplements, your doctor will be able see the changes, and see your determination. If he or she still resists, I suggest you get another doctor—one who has your best interests in mind. I'll talk in more detail about the dangers of some of the heart disease drugs so popular in America later in the book.

The single biggest factor contributing to heart disease in America is our poor diet. We eat too much fat, too many processed foods, and not enough fresh vegetables. In the 1950s, the Japanese diet was 16 percent fat and they had almost no incidence of heart disease. Today their diet is 26 percent fat and heart disease is the second leading cause of death in Japan. In the U.S. the average diet contains 36–40 percent fat.

I feel that cholesterol and high blood pressure are way overrated as risk factors for heart disease. I haven't even included chapters on them in this book because if you follow these 22 steps I can virtually guarantee that your blood pressure and cholesterol will automatically fall! Such risk factors as low antioxidant status or high homocysteine are more telling, but the American public hasn't heard about them because they don't sell drugs. Selling drugs to lower high blood pressure and cholesterol is a *billion*-dollar industry, yet the evidence that these drugs actually lower your chances of dying from heart disease is extremely skimpy.

A major study published in JAMA (*Journal of the Ameri-*

can Medical Association) proves my point. This huge trial began in 1958 and included more than 12,000 men in seven different countries, including the United States, Japan and five European countries. Total cholesterol was measured in men ages 40 through 59 years of age and followed up at five- to ten-year intervals. Blood pressure, diet, deaths from heart disease, and a variety of other lifestyle factors such as cigarette smoking, were also tracked.

Although statistically there was a weak relationship between high cholesterol levels and heart disease, there was a far stronger relationship between diet and heart disease. From country to country, the rate of death from heart disease varied, and cholesterol levels varied, but the variation was not at all proportional to cholesterol levels. In other words, those with the highest cholesterol levels did not necessarily have the highest rates of heart disease. For example, in Japan, Southern Europe and the Mediterranean, the rate of death from heart disease did not rise significantly even when blood cholesterol levels went as high as 250 milligrams per deciliter. Death rates *did* rise in the U.S. and northern Europe with cholesterol, especially when cholesterol went over 250 mg/dL.

What was striking was that cultures eating less meat and more fish, fruits and vegetables, and drinking more wine, had significantly lower rates of death from heart disease. Furthermore, there was a strong correlation between diets high in polyunsaturated fatty acids (vegetable oils prone to oxidation/rancidity) and a high rate of death from heart disease (more about that later), and correspondingly less death in those cultures that ate more monounsaturated fats such as olive oil.

Those countries with the highest intake of antioxidants and bioflavonoids had the lowest death rates from heart disease, with Japan having a much higher intake and a much lower rate of death than any of the other countries.

You're probably aware that cigarette smoking is known as the major preventable risk factor for cardiovascular disease. I think poor nutrition, lack of exercise, too much stress, an overload of environmental toxins, and a long list of prescription drugs should also be known as preventable risk factors. In each chapter, we'll talk about these less well-known risk factors, and I'll give you simple, specific, practical methods for lowering your risk of heart disease.

The estimated cost for cardiovascular disease in 1994 by the American Heart Association was 128 billion dollars. This includes the cost of physicians and nursing services, hospital and nursing home services, the cost of medications and loss of productivity. But the personal cost of heart disease is the biggest loss of all because the heart is irreplaceable. Let's work together now for a healthy, vibrant, energetic life at all ages!

CHAPTER 1

Cut Back on the Sweets

Kicking the sugar habit is one of the simplest and most effective steps you can take to prevent heart disease. Americans have the highest rate of heart disease in the world, and I believe our overindulgence in sugar, combined with poor nutrition and lack of exercise, is the single biggest cause of heart disease.

I strongly recommend you keep your sugar intake low. For some people, that means not eating it at all, because just a little sugar leads to eating a lot of sugar. Others can have something sweet a couple of times a week and leave it at that. If you fall into the first category, you're best off just avoiding sugar altogether unless it comes in a piece of fruit.

A study of rats and lifespan published in the *Journal of Clinical Nutrition* illustrates just how detrimental sugar is. One group of rats was given access to a diet that was 66 percent sugar, and the other group was fed a normal diet. The rats fed sugar water had a significantly shorter lifespan.

Here's a partial list of what sugar does to your body:

- Creates drowsiness and mental sluggishness.
- Suppresses the immune system.
- Generates free radicals.
- Contributes to obesity.
- Upsets glucose and insulin balance.
- Can contribute to diabetes.
- Causes hypoglycemia with its symptoms of fatigue, irritability and weakness.
- Contributes to candidiasis, an overgrowth of yeast in the body.
- Raises triglycerides, a type of blood fat associated with heart disease.
- Damages the kidneys.
- Contributes to gallstones by raising cholesterol content of bile.
- Causes premature aging.
- Upsets the acid balance in the stomach.
- Contributes to arthritis.
- Can increase cholesterol.
- Interferes with the utilization of protein.

- Makes food allergies worse.
- Sorbitol causes diarrhea and irritable bowel syndrome in some people.

Sugar depletes or interferes with the absorption of:

- Vitamin C
- B-complex vitamins
- Chromium
- Copper
- Calcium
- Magnesium

All of these nutrients are vital to the proper functioning of your heart and circulatory system. Since the average person in America eats 133 pounds of sweeteners a year, and the average American teenager eats 300 pounds of sugar a year, it should come as no surprise that we have an epidemic of heart diease. Some 20 to 25 percent of our daily calories are consumed in sugar.

WHY DO WE LOVE SUGAR SO MUCH?

Sugar quickly and temporarily raises our blood sugar, which stimulates the adrenal glands and creates a "high." The body has a built-in sugar regulator, but it isn't designed to handle the intense concentrations of sugar we get when we eat a pastry or drink a soda. To give you an example of just how far from Mother Nature a soft drink is, you would have to eat 30 yards of sugar cane to get the sugar you get in one can of Coca Cola. This is the equivalent of nine teaspoons of sugar. As designed by nature, fruit and sugar cane come packed with fiber and nutrients, which you get none of when you eat the refined version.

You're probably familiar with that rush of energy, or sense of well-being after you eat sugar. But within half an hour to an hour after eating sugar, your blood sugar plummets. This signals the brain to turn on the adrenal glands, which try to get the blood sugar back up, but in the process adrenaline is released too. Andrenaline is the substance that, when we lived in caves, gave us the "fight or flight" response. It's our way of coping with a sudden fright or stress. Our heart beats faster, our blood pressure rises, our muscles prepare for action and our blood leaves our digestive system for other more survival-oriented parts of our body. When this happens regularly, the adrenal glands become exhausted.

As your body works extra hard to pump its heavy sugar load out of the blood it will overreact, pump too much out, and blood sugar often ends up below what it was before we ate the sugar. This plunge, along with the adrenaline surge, can cause fatigue, weakness, shakiness, dizziness, "spaciness," headaches and irritability. So we reach for more sugar to get our blood sugar back up, and pretty soon we're looking for our next sugar fix every hour or so. Meanwhile, the precipitous rise and fall of our blood sugar has a chain reaction all over the body, causing imbalances ranging from too much acid in the stomach to too much cholesterol in the bile, and the depletion of essential vitamins and minerals.

KICKING THE HABIT

Sugar is hard to get away from in our culture. I know many mothers who have very good intentions about not letting their kids get hooked on sugar, but who give up because it's so difficult to keep it out of their diet. Children get sugar from day care on through kindergarten and grade school; they get it when they go over to play at another child's house, at birthday parties and in many types of processed food. Pretty soon the clamoring for sugary foods is constant, and most parents just get worn down. Sugar in and of itself is not a bad food—but in the amounts we give it to our children and ourselves, it is destructive.

The best way to kick sugar out of your life is to start reading labels. Many low fat foods substitute a lot of sugar or salt. Be aware. Sugar goes under lots of names, but it's all still sugar. "Ose" at the end of a word stands for sugar. There's sucrose (common table sugar), dextrose, and fructose (fruit sugar). Watch out for highly refined fructose, or high fructose corn syrup, which is used in cola drinks and many of the so-called natural soft drinks such as Snapple. There's nothing natural about them because they're so concentrated. Brown sugar is also not healthier for you, contrary to popular opinion. It's just white sugar with molasses coloring. If you give up processed foods, which I'll talk more about later, it will be much easier to avoid sugar.

Another hidden source of sugar is alcohol. Most alcohol contains sugar, and many people who drink too much are also sugarholics. If you want to kick the sugar habit, you would be wise to give up alcohol, at least for a month or so, to get your body out of the sugar rut. If and when you decide to drink alcohol again, be alert to whether your sugar cravings return.

There are studies showing that sugar does less harm when you get plenty of exercise. Sugar is a calorie that is burned off quickly when you exercise, so if you do have a sweet, be sure to burn it off!

If you have a sweet tooth, have some fruit. Grapes are especially sweet. Apples and pears make good afternoon snacks. Although the sugars in fruit are still sugar, they aren't absorbed as quickly as refined white sugar, and unlike white sugar, which has no nutritional value, a piece of fruit has vitamins, minerals and fiber. (If you have a craving for chocolate, you may be deficient in magnesium—try munching on some figs or almonds.) When you get an afternoon or evening craving for fat, try a handful of unsalted nuts such as almonds or cashews. But don't overdo it—nuts are packed with calories!

CHAPTER 2

Cut Back on the Fats

The promotion of margarine and partially hydrogenated vegetable oils as "heart-healthy" oils is one of the biggest lies ever foisted on the American public. I believe our consumption of these "fake fats," along with sugar, is one of the major reasons America has the highest rate of heart disease in the world.

Contrary to the doctrines of popular diet fads, fat is not inherently bad for you. However, all fat is bad for you in excess. Some fat is essential to good health. Fats aren't there just to add to your waistline, they are an essential part of the make-up of every cell in the body and participate in nearly every bodily function. A balanced diet will include all the types of fats found in nature in varying amounts, and will avoid the refined and manmade fats.

The most important key concerning fats is to keep your fat calories low: no more than 25 percent of your total daily calories, and I keep mine around 20 percent.

For most Americans, sticking to this rule means cutting fat intake by half. I don't want you to deprive yourself, but I do want you to become *aware* of the fats in your diet, and gradually work to reduce the amount and replace the unhealthy fats with healthy fats.

For example, the amount of fat the average adult would want to eat in a day would be 30 to 40 grams. (Growing children can eat up to 30 percent of their calories in fat.) A tablespoon of butter contains 12 grams of fat. An ounce of sharp cheddar cheese contains 9 grams. A 3½ ounce portion of sirloin steak contains 13 grams of fat. If you don't have a sense of how much fat your diet contains, buy one of the many books now available that lists the fat content of nearly every type of food available in North America. Once you have a sense of how much fat you're eating every day, put the book on the shelf and focus on changing how you eat.

BUSTING THE AMERICAN FAT MYTHS

It may surprise you when I tell you that saturated fat is not bad for you. It is *too much* saturated fat that is bad for you. You only need small quantities of saturated fat in your diet to be healthy.

Saturated fat is found in the highest concentrations in red meat, butter, coconut oil and other tropical oils. They are also found in smaller concentrations (6 to 20 percent) in all oils. Saturated fats are easy to digest, and we burn them up as energy quickly and efficiently. If you exercise a lot, you can afford to eat more saturated fats.

The total amount of saturated fat in your diet can range from as low as 2 percent of your total calories, up to about 10 percent, or half your total fat intake.

While it is true that an *excess* of saturated fat can contribute to heart disease, let's not go overboard in trying to eliminate saturated fat from our diets. The studies cited to back up the prevailing belief that saturated fat is bad for you are very faulty. Those studies done with tropical oil consumption (coconut oil, palm oil) were done with refined oils. Those populations around the world that consume saturated tropical oils are eating unrefined oils in relatively small amounts, and they are quite healthy and free of heart disease.

Another error in these studies is not comparing *total* fat intake to the amount of saturated fat eaten. In other words, no study has been done that I'm aware of on people whose total fat intake is only 20 percent, but who eat a high percentage of that 20 percent in saturated fat. Other factors not taken into account in the saturated fat studies are the amount of exercise; amount of refined sugars and flours in the diet; amount of fiber, fresh fruits and vegetables in the diet; amount of trans-fatty acids in the diet, and stress levels. All of these factors weigh heavily in heart disease. My advice on saturated fat is to go ahead and include some in your diet, just don't overdo it.

CHAPTER 3

Eat Healthy Fats and Oils

Now that we've busted some of America's fat myths, let's take a look at how the various oils and fats fare on the "heart-healthy" scale. Most of our information about

how fats and oils react in the body is based on population
studies rather than direct biochemical knowledge. In
other words, we know that populations eating lots of olive
oil have healthier hearts, but we're not sure exactly why.
Although we know a lot about the molecular structure
of fats and oils, we know surprisingly little about what
they do once they're in the body. One thing we do know
for sure is that rancid fats or oils are unhealthy.

OLIVE OIL IS HEART-HEALTHY

Olive oil is a monounsaturated fat, which tends to be
stable (it doesn't go rancid easily). Many studies have
shown that populations consuming high amounts of olive
oil tend to have much lower rates of heart disease. Mono
unsaturated oils are also found in canola oil, peanuts,
almonds, pistachios, pecans, hazelnuts, cashews, macada
mia nuts, and avocados.

Although peanut oil is fairly stable, peanuts are highly
susceptible to a type of fungus containing aflatoxins
which are poisonous, and it also tends to be a crop heav
ily sprayed with pesticides and fungicides. I don't recom
mend peanut oil unless it's organic and from a highly
reputable source.

Olive and canola oil are the most stable of the mono
unsaturated oils, and the healthiest. If you buy canola oi
not preserved with vitamin E, please open a 400 IU cap
sule of vitamin E and put the contents in the bottle.

Olive oil is the most stable of the monounsaturated
oils, and a high consumption of it has been shown to
actually lower heart disease. It's very important to re
member, however, that the Italians and Greeks consum
ing this oil at such a high rate are eating *unrefined* olive
oil. Refined olive oil will not have the same benefits
because most of the nutrients are taken out of it, includ
ing and especially vitamin E. Please buy unrefined virgin
olive oil and if you can get it, organic. In fact, all of the

oils you buy should be unrefined. The refining process uses toxic solvents and takes all the goodness out of the oil.

AVOID THE UNSATURATED OILS

With the exception of canola oil, which is partially refined, I recommend that as a general rule you avoid all unsaturated, polyunsaturated, hydrogenated and partially hydrogenated oils. This means that for the most part you need to avoid vegetable oils unless you can find them unrefined and very fresh, or preserved with vitamin E and in a lightproof container.

Vegetable oils, also called polyunsaturated and super polyunsaturated oils, have caused most of the confusion about oils. Unrefined, very freshly pressed vegetable oils are a wonderful food, and our ancestors often had them delivered weekly from the town oil vendor. They were delivered weekly, along with milk and other spoilable products because, being unsaturated, these oils are very unstable and thus go rancid very easily, especially when exposed to light and air. Rancid oils create chain reactions of oxidation in the body, setting loose free radicals that do damage to cells, causing disease and aging. To avoid rancidity these days, manufacturers heavily refine vegetable oils, which strips away their nutrients and adds the residues of toxic chemical solvents.

The most common manufacturing method for preventing rancidity is hydrogenation. This process adds hydrogen to unsaturated oils, making them more saturated and thus more stable. You might think this is good, because it prevents rancidity, but these manmade semisaturated fats are not found in nature, so your body doesn't know what to do with them. Total hydrogenation creates a solid fat such as margarine or shortening. These so-called trans-fatty acids have been heavily implicated in heart disease. I believe they may also be responsible for many of our chronic diseases. Please stay away from them!

I realize that highly unstable oils such as flax oil are very popular right now, but I suggest using them in moderation, and only if you believe you are deficient in essential fatty acids (EFAs), because they are so susceptible to rancidity.

Use your daily allotment of fat calories wisely, by consuming nutrient rich, unprocessed and unrefined fats and oils as we find them in nature. Our bodies only need tiny amounts of EFAs, so if you eat plenty of fresh, unprocessed fruits and vegetables, you will get all your body needs.

Fish Oil Is Heart-healthy

Fish oil contains omega-3 fatty acids, unsaturated oils that seem to help prevent heart disease. The body can also make the omega-3s from alpha-linolenic acid (an essential fatty acid found in flax oil, and in smaller amounts in canola oil, pumpkin seeds, soybeans, walnuts and dark green vegetables).

Omega-3 fatty acids reduce blood clotting without the risk of too much bleeding or hemorrhaging; they lower blood pressure; improve blood flow; and over time can aid in the process of removing cholesterol from the blood and fatty deposits from the arteries. The omega-3s are also a precursor to prostaglandins, important hormonelike substances that regulate many body functions.

Good fish sources of omega-3s include salmon, herring, mackerel, tuna, sardines and wild trout. Omega-3s are also found in spirulina, an algae grown in fresh water. If you take fish oil supplements, be sure they come from deep, northern waters, they are unrefined, and have been preserved in some way to prevent rancidity.

Omega-3s used to be found in beef, back in the days when cattle grazed on native grasses and plants instead of being stuffed with corn, other fattening grains and estrogen in feed lots. This may be one reason our ancestors could eat plenty of meat in their diet and not suffer from heart disease. (Believe me, unprocessed foods, fiber and exercise made a difference too!) It is becoming increasingly common to find range-fed beef in health food stores and even some supermarkets. Ask around for it.

CHAPTER 4

Eat More Fresh, Whole Foods and Fewer Processed Foods

You are what you eat, but if you eat a lot of refined foods you won't be a more refined person, you will be a drastically less healthy person! Our national health began a dramatic decline when refined and processed foods were introduced. The rise of chronic degenerative diseases such as heart disease and diabetes has risen along with the rise in consumption of foods that have all the nutrients stripped out of them and harmful preservatives and additives put back in. If you're eating lots of canned, packaged, preserved and frozen foods, I'd like you to gradually begin switching to whole foods. As a bonus, when you fill up on fresh vegetables and fruits, you are likely to eat fewer fats and sweets. Fresh foods are also easier on your wallet. Processed and packaged foods cost more while providing you with less nutrition.

Foods packaged by nature come complete with all the nutrients you need. When I talk about whole foods I mean essentially as nature made them. You get enzymes, vitamins, minerals, amino acids and hundreds of other nutritional substances you need for a healthy, energetic body capable of handling stress and fighting off disease.

Go for the Whole Grains and Legumes

Grains such as wheat, corn, millet, barley, oats, quinoa, amaranth and rice are not only delicious, they contain a wonderful potpourri of nutrients, as well as fiber. I'd like you to get reacquainted with whole grains. Try oatmeal or a whole grain cereal or bread for breakfast. For lunch, have a salad on a bed of brown rice or millet. Add barley to soups and stews, and try some corn tortillas with your vegetables. Add whole grains, which are complex carbohydrates, to your diet gradually. If you switch suddenly your digestive system may protest with gas and bloating.

Whole Foods Are Your Ticket to a Healthy Heart

People who eat plenty of fresh vegetables and fruits have a lower cancer risk, as well as less heart disease and a lower risk of diabetes. Instead of buying the canned and frozen varieties of vegetables and fruits, head for the produce section. Treat yourself and your family to daily salads, lightly steamed vegetables seasoned with olive oil and lemon, and a delicious dessert of fresh fruit. Not only will you live longer, you'll feel better along the way.

FIBER IS A HEART PROTECTOR

When you eat whole foods you get lots of fiber. Fiber is a plant substance that is not digested. You've probably heard a lot about how good fiber is for you. Well, it's true. The American Cancer Institute recommends 25 to 30 grams of fiber a day, and yet most people only get half of that. I'd like you to get 30 grams, or approximately 1 ounce of fiber every day, and here's why. Fiber speeds up the movement of food through the intestinal tract. The faster the food moves through, the less time there is for your body to absorb fats. Fiber also acts like a whisk broom that sweeps the small intestine clean, keeping it free of infection, and in the large colon it absorbs the toxins being removed from the body.

The good news is that increasing your fiber is a piece of cake (so to speak). If you're eating whole foods and plenty of fresh vegetables, it's easy to get your fiber every day. If you're over the age of 50 and need a little help, you can add anywhere from 1 teaspoon to 1 tablespoon of psyllium seed or psyllium husk (pronounced silly-um) to your diet daily. You know this fiber as Metamucil, but unfortunately Metamucil has a lot of sugar or artificial sweeteners. Pure psyllium is better for you and it's cheaper. You can buy psyllium in health food stores in bulk one-pound or two-pound containers.

Psyllium is easy to use. Just stir it into juice or water and drink immediately. Then drink a glass of water immediately afterward. (You can count these toward your 6 to 10 glasses of water per day.) Be sure to drink plenty of water. Start with a teaspoon of psyllium, and if necessary work your way up gradually to a tablespoon.

If you have a bowel disorder, check with a physician first before using psyllium or increasing the fiber in your diet. It's important to add fiber to your diet gradually if you're not used to it, or you could experience gas and bloating.

THERE'S GOOD CHEMISTRY
IN FRESH, WHOLE FOODS

Fruits and vegetables are excellent sources of antioxidants, which are your number one defense against the damage done to your blood vessels by free radicals. Cruciferous vegetables such as broccoli, cauliflower and cabbage contain dithiolthiones, thiocyanates, isothiocyanates, and sulforaphane, which stimulate the production of enzymes such as glutathione which is also an antioxidant. Other substances found in fruits and vegetables, such as polyphenols, folic acid, minerals and chlorophyll, also work to keep your heart healthy.

In whole grains you get vitamin E, some of the B vitamins, and compounds called phenols, yet another form of antioxidant. Other compounds in grains, including lignans, flavonoids and phytic acid, also contribute to a healthy heart.

An extensive survey of studies of 19 Western European and five non-European countries of heart disease and lifestyle showed that men were far less likely to die prematurely of heart disease if their intake of vegetables was high. The strongest association showed up in vegetables that contain vitamin E.

CHAPTER 5

Use Alcohol in Moderation

Caution and moderation are the watchwords for drinking alcohol. Studies show that a low alcohol intake, particularly of red wine, does protect against heart disease when included as part of a healthy diet. However, even just a bit too much alcohol can bump up blood pressure and help create nutritional deficiencies which increase your risk of heart disease.

EXCESS ALCOHOL RAISES BLOOD PRESSURE

It's well documented that alcohol can be associated with high blood pressure. Supporting evidence comes from studies like one from Belgium, which looked at lifestyle and blood pressure and found that increased alcohol intake led to higher diastolic and systolic blood pressure readings in 405 men and 379 women. Keep alcohol intake down and you're helping to keep the lid on hypertension and therefore heart disease, too.

ALCOHOLISM AND HEART DISEASE

Alcoholics have a greatly increased risk of cardiovascular disease. Chronic alcoholics frequently suffer a deficiency of magnesium, which could have a causative link with heart disease. This was the finding of research done at the University of California Medical Center. For details on magnesium's importance to heart health, see the chapter on magnesium.

LOW ALCOHOL FOR LOWER RISK

A study published in the *New England Journal of Medicine* investigated alcohol consumption and mortality in over 85,000 women ranging in age from 34 to 59, without a history of cancer or heart disease. Heavy drinking was associated with increased risks of death from cancer and cirrhosis of the liver. Light to moderate drinkers (1.5 to 29.9 grams per day), however, were found to have a slightly lower death rate than non-drinkers. Furthermore, this low to moderate intake was of most benefit to women over 50, and women with risk factors for heart disease. The message coming from the scientific evidence is that a little alcohol can be beneficial, but even just a little too much is bad for you.

EAT WELL, DRINK WISELY FOR A HAPPY HEART

Why do the French suffer less heart disease despite the relatively high consumption of animal fats? This is known in scientific circles as "the French paradox." You may have read media hype about wine as a magical heart elixir. In fact, the real story isn't so simple.

The French paradox was investigated in a review of heart disease rates, alcohol consumption, diet and death rates in 21 relatively affluent countries. While the study did find that wine does seem to protect against heart disease, drinking more did not increase protection. Interestingly, the study also found lower rates of heart disease in geographical areas where larger amounts of fruit were consumed, indicating that the health benefits didn't rest with wine alone. It was also found that whatever the protection provided by drinking wine, people in France did not live longer as a result. In fact, the French have one of the highest rates of liver disease in the world.

More light on the subject comes from a Harvard School of Public Health study which looked specifically at alcohol in the Mediterranean diet. The study found that the Mediterranean diet typically includes one or two drinks per day and large amounts of fruit, vegetables and grains. The researchers concluded that this kind of responsible consumption of alcohol does appear to reduce the risk of cardiovascular disease.

RED WINE IS BEST

Components of red wine can reduce the activity of clotting agents in the blood. This was a conclusion of an animal study reported in the *Medical Tribune*. This could help to explain the protective effect of low alcohol intake. Red wine, white wine and ethanol all produced a reduction in blood clotting tendencies in rats. As soon as the doses were stopped, though, levels in the rats fed on ethanol or white wine shot up dramatically, especially in those given ethanol. Clotting activity stayed low, however, in the rats given red wine. Researchers believe either tannins or polyphenols could be the compounds in red wine that produce this effect. Whatever the particular chemistry, red wine is the preferred form of alcohol for heart-protective effects.

CHAPTER 6

Eat More Garlic

Garlic is the herb of legend and myth. It is mentioned in the Bible, in Homer's *Odyssey* and in ancient Chinese texts, and has been found in the tombs of ancient Egyptians. Now we have dozens of scientific studies to back up most of the claims for garlic's prowess in keeping us healthy.

While garlic may or may not work to ward off vampires, it does a great job at neutralizing three risk factors for heart disease—high blood fats, high blood pressure, and blood clotting.

Some 2000 recent studies by the world's top researchers have established that garlic could have a real impact on the most serious modern diseases, heart disease included. A University of Western Oregon study of diet in 15 countries showed rates of heart disease were lower in those with higher garlic consumption.

GETTING CHOLESTEROL DOWN WITH GARLIC

Although it's known that cutting down on excessive amounts of high-cholesterol food can help lower LDL cholesterol levels in the blood, more than 70 percent of cholesterol is made inside the body. Cholesterol is essential for the production of all your steroid hormones, including your sex hormones. Garlic helps to keep the production of cholesterol in healthy balance. It slows down internal cholesterol production as well as cutting the negative effects of too much dietary cholesterol.

Rats whose diets were supplemented with garlic extract for two months had significantly lower blood cholesterol, less fat in their tissues and less cholesterol and fat in their livers. In another study, rats on a high-cholesterol diet supplemented with garlic had LDL levels nearly identical to those rats on a cholesterol-free diet.

One study of a vegetarian community in India found that the members eating liberal amounts of garlic and onions averaged 25 percent lower cholesterol levels and 50 percent lower blood fats than those who didn't eat garlic and onions. Subsequent studies support these findings. One, reported in the *American Journal of Clinical Nutrition*, showed that out of the 62 patients in the study, the 31 given a placebo showed little change in their cholesterol levels. But heart disease patients given garlic oil daily for ten months enjoyed a steady decrease in LDL levels together with a progressive increase in levels of HDL cholesterol, which is protective against heart disease.

A study at California's Loma Linda University School of Medicine gave 32 people with high cholesterol levels aged garlic extract for six months. The study was nearly abandoned when patients given the extract at first saw their blood fat levels rise! However, after the intial rise, LDL levels steadily dropped, with the benefit, too, that HDL levels rose. These findings led the researchers to conclude that garlic inhibits LDL production. The initial rise in blood fat levels also indicated that garlic helps to move stored fats from tissues into the bloodstream, helping them eventually to be eliminated.

It may be that the sulfur compounds in garlic inhibit the activity of a key enzyme that initiates cholesterol synthesis. This kind of chemistry helps garlic keep heart disease at bay.

GARLIC UNDOES HEART DISEASE DAMAGE

Studies by Dr. Arun Bordia, a cardiologist at Tagore Medical College in India, have revealed that regular garlic consumption not only helps arteries stay clear, but also reduces the degree of artery blockage. The reversal of atherosclerosis has actually been measured in rabbits fed on a diet supplemented with garlic.

Heart disease patients have seen the benefits, too. Dr. Bordia conducted a study of 432 patients over three years. Half ate garlic daily and half ate none. Those not eating garlic saw no real cardiovascular changes. But blood cholesterol and blood pressure dropped by about 10 percent in the garlic eaters, who also experienced less angina. Most dramatic of all, deaths among the garlic eaters dropped by 50 percent in the second year and by 66 percent in the third.

GARLIC STOPS THE CLOTS

Ancient folklore has long seen garlic used as a blood tonic—even for horses! Now science has proved the old remedies true. Researchers have discovered four powerful anti-clotting agents in garlic, at least one of which is a more effective anticoagulant than aspirin.

German studies at Saarland University in Homburg/Saar have demonstrated how garlic compounds help blood clots dissolve faster and improve blood fluidity. A report from the University of Wisconsin has shown how aged garlic extract supplementation inhibits the production of a blood clot trigger. And 50 medical students in India recently saw their blood clotting time and clot dissolving activity improve by about 20 percent after eating three raw garlic cloves a day.

Coronary thrombosis is the condition in which a blood clot forms in an artery leading to the heart. It can result in myocardial infarction or heart attack. Eating garlic to help prevent the thrombosis in the first place makes good sense.

GARLIC LOWERS BLOOD PRESSURE

Experts estimate that as many as 20 percent of Americans suffer from hypertension, or high blood pressure. As a major risk factor for cardiovascular disease, it is widely treated with drugs. However, most blood pressure medication causes moderate to severe side effects. These can be avoided by simply including the drugs naturally available in plants like garlic.

Garlic has been a hypertension treatment for centuries in China and Japan. It's also widely used today in Germany. In fact, tests were recently performed on a German over-the-counter garlic preparation. A dose equivalent to two daily garlic cloves reduced blood pressure in patients with mild hypertension. The garlic produced a blood pressure reduction over the three-month study, showing that garlic may even have a cumulative effect in the body.

A variety of studies involving animals and humans, conducted over the past seven decades, show that garlic lowers blood pressure. Studies on people with diagnosed hypertension as far afield as China and Bulgaria have shown that garlic in various forms produces a fall in blood pressure.

Animal studies show garlic relaxes the smooth muscles of blood vessels. Another blood pressure-lowering mechanism was reported in the German scientific journal *Planta Medica*. It seems that a small garlic peptide inhibits the production of a blood pressure-raising hormone. Whatever the mechanisms, science and history both provide strong evidence that garlic lowers blood pressure.

How to Take Garlic?

Raw garlic has been shown to be beneficial, but it's also true that eating it can have side effects like nausea, vomiting and diarrhea, and very large intake can damage red blood cells. Many beneficial garlic compounds are actually produced when it is cut, crushed or heated. Although these processes cause the loss of allicin, a powerful germ-killing substance, research found that allicin kills beneficial as well as harmful cells indiscriminately. Supplemental garlic oil often contains only a small fraction of garlic because it is mixed with other vegetable oils and consists only of the garlic chemicals distilled at high temperatures.

After raw garlic, the most effective form of garlic appears to be aged extract of organic garlic, but they all have some beneficial effects.

CHAPTER 7

Eat More Soy

The death rate from heart disease in Japan is roughly half the rate in the United States. There are many studies showing how diet plays a key role behind the statistics on heart disease. In the famous Ni-Hon-San Study, re searchers found that men eating a traditional Japanese diet had the lowest rate of heart disease. Men who moved to Honolulu, and ate a more Western-style diet had a higher rate of heart disease. But the highest death rate from heart disease fell to the Japanese men in San Francisco consuming a typical American diet.

Studies show that a diet high in harmful fats is a major risk factor for heart disease. Because soy contains "good" fats, and tends to be lower in fat than food from animal sources, it's a good source of protein. In addition, researchers have shown how isolated compounds in soy may directly prevent heart disease by altering blood fat levels. Extensive research reveals that it produces a range of effects that are highly valuable in the control and prevention of heart disease.

SOY IS A CHOLESTEROL BUSTER

In Italy, the government is so convinced of the value of soy that soy protein is provided free of charge to doctors treating patients with high cholesterol levels. Research shows that Italian men and women aged 33 to 44 years of age with serum cholesterol levels below 220 mg/dl have five times less risk of developing coronary artery disease than those with levels of 256 mg/dl or over.

It is believed that soy may have antioxidant properties in the body, which would explain why it decreases the production of "bad" oxidized LDL cholesterol. In one interesting study by Japanese researchers from Hirosaki University School of Medicine, soy milk was added to the diet of rabbits. The results found soy to be even more effective at lowering unhealthy cholesterol levels than Probucol, a commercial antioxidant supplement.

A University of Illinois study looked at 26 men with elevated cholesterol levels who were put on a low-fat, low-cholesterol diet. Over a four-month period, the men substituted half their normal protein intake with soy products or nonfat dried milk. Soy protein gave the best results, producing significant cholesterol level reductions with just 50 grams per day. Results from studies in Milan tell the same success story, showing that even when cholesterol is deliberately added to a diet including soy products, soy continues to cut cholesterol levels.

The studies make it clear that by cutting "bad" cholesterol levels, soy makes a powerful addition to a heart disease prevention diet.

Some studies show that blood glucagon levels rise after soy protein consumption. Glucagon is a hormone released by the pancreas. Researchers speculate that a shift in glucagon levels may alter the activity of an enzyme needed by the body to manufacture cholesterol. This is the way a drug, Mevacor, works in lowering cholesterol. Soy may well do the same thing naturally.

Animal studies show that as well as lowering cholesterol levels, soy produces an increase in blood plasma levels of thyroxine, a hormone produced by the thyroid gland. Interestingly, the rise in thyroxine always precedes the drop in cholesterol. Sure enough, people with underactive thyroid glands tend to have high levels of blood cholesterol. This leads researchers to believe that soy somehow stimulates thyroxene production, which in turn lowers blood cholesterol.

PHYTOESTROGENS BLOCK CHOLESTEROL

After menopause, estrogen levels drop in women, and cholesterol levels typically rise, bringing an increased risk of coronary artery disease. Some researchers theorize that estrogen decreases the amount of LDL circulating in the blood by increasing the number of LDL receptors in cells. Soy is high in phytoestrogens, which occupy estrogen receptor sites, producing a weak, but effective estrogen response in the body without the cancer-stimulating effects of estrogen. Researchers theorize that soy's estrogenic activity could well be linked to its cholesterol-lowering ability.

SOY IS A CHEMICAL POWERHOUSE

Genistein is a substance unique to soy which has been shown to inhibit cell growth and migration, particularly in tumors. Scientists speculate that genistein may work in the same way to prevent the growth of cells which form plaque deposits in arteries.

Phytic acid, also found in soy, binds to iron and increases copper absorption in the body. Copper deficiency, in several studies, has been associated with high cholesterol. Researchers suggest, too, that soy binds with bile, which is then excreted in the feces. This promotes the production of more bile salts, a process that uses up cholesterol and so reduces levels in the blood stream.

Studies show that another chemical, the amino acid lysine, increases LDL levels when added to a soy diet. Lysine and other amino acids are at lower levels in soy than in animal protein. This leads scientists to believe that soy's particular mix of amino acids may help to prevent the formation of plaque. Indeed, it's clear that soy's overall chemical make-up makes it a frontline food in heart disease prevention.

INCLUDING SOY IN YOUR DIET

Soy products are made from soybeans processed in various ways, including soaking, fermenting, grinding, sprouting and frying. You can choose from soy milk, tofu, tempeh, miso, soy flour and sauce, although soy sauce is high in sodium and contains the least nutrients. There are many possible ways to include soy in every meal. I like to make shakes with soy protein powder. Always be sure to include soy as part of a complete low-fat, whole food, vitamin rich, high-fiber diet.

CHAPTER 8

Drink Plenty of Clean Water

Water is your top heart-healthy drink, in a class by itself. Nothing else comes close to clean water's lack of toxicity, safety and ability to keep your biochemistry whirring smoothly along. It has no calories, no caffeine, no sugar, no additives or preservatives, and no fat. Some 60 percent of the human body is water, and you need plenty of it every day to stay healthy and flush out toxins. Water is more necessary for sustaining life than food. You can survive more than a month without food, but not more than a few days without water.

I recommend everyone drink six to 10 glasses of clean water daily. The amount you drink will depend on your body weight, height, biochemistry and your lifestyle. If you are exercising heavily, pregnant or nursing, you will need significantly more water. Running a marathon on a hot day can deplete the body of as much as six quarts of water. A bicycle racer climbing hills can lose up to three quarts an hour.

Dehydration while doing vigorous exercise can cause the heartbeat to accelerate abnormally. Chronic dehydration can increase your risk of heart attack and stroke. A study done in Denmark showed that postoperative stroke patients who became dehydrated had a much greater risk of having a second stroke. Another study done in Italy on older men who had a heart attack showed that over half of them were dehydrated. Dehydration can also cause abnormal heartbeats, constipation, urinary tract infections, kidney stones, immune deficiencies, electrolyte imbalances, skin problems, and most likely contributes to many chronic diseases, including arthritis and heart disease. It's so simple to drink plenty of clean water that nobody should subject themselves to this heart attack risk.

Clean water is one of your body's primary weapons against free radical damage caused by toxins. Blood and lymphatic fluid, which carry nutrients into cells and toxins out, are primarily made up of water. Water is essential for good digestion and elimination of toxins through sweat and urine. Because water is a solvent, it helps rid your bloodstream of excess fat, which can help to reduce your blood serum cholesterol level.

Avoid Tap Water

Drinking plenty of water can do your heart more harm than good if it's not pure and clean. Chlorine and fluoride have been clearly implicated in a range of illnesses, including heart disease. Chlorine changes the way the body metabolizes fats, raising LDL cholesterol and lowering HDL cholesterol, the opposite effect of what you need to keep your arteries clean and clear. Communities with high levels of fluoride in their tap water have significantly higher rates of death from heart disease.

Cleaning Up Your Water Act

I recommend you buy bottled water or even better, use a filtration system. You can purchase an inexpensive water filter or a complete household unit, depending on your needs and your budget. The least expensive route is a pitcher with a filter attached. All you do is pour the water through. Ideally I'd like to see you with a more sophisticated filtration system in your home that eliminates heavy metals, chlorine, benzene and other carcinogens. Prices start around $200 and you can easily install sink-top units yourself.

Water filtration companies can install water filtration units in your home. Many companies have units large enough to serve a whole house, apartment, or condominium, and others small enough to fit under or even above the kitchen sink. Shop around for the best price. Ask for an analysis of what remains in your water after it has been filtered.

There are currently three types of water filtration systems that eliminate most pollutants from your water. One combines reverse osmosis with carbon filters. Another uses a zinc/copper and charcoal filter, and the third is a ceramic filter. Check your local telephone book under Water Filtration to find companies that sell these systems.

These systems enable you to filter your tap water for pennies a gallon. It tastes great, which makes it easy for you to drink the 6 to 10 glasses I recommend. If you like to drink cold water, store some in the refrigerator. That way you'll always have available a cold, delicious, thirst-quenching beverage with no calories.

CHAPTER 9

Pass on the Salt

Sodium, or salt, is one of our most important minerals—we're not healthy without it. Sodium is a metallic element that becomes part of our body chemistry when it combines with other elements such as chloride. Table salt is sodium chloride, or NaCl.

The following is a list of salt's most important functions in the body:

- It aids in keeping calcium and other minerals soluble in the blood.
- It helps regulate muscle contractions.
- It plays a part in nerve stimulation.
- It plays an important role in maintaining fluid balance in the cells.
- It is necessary for the production of hydrochloric acid in the stomach.
- It helps regulate fluid balance when the temperature rises.

Since the average American consumes about 15 pounds of sodium each year—this amounts to a daily intake of about 60 times what is required by the body—we hardly need to worry about getting too much. Our need for salt will vary according to our weight, diet, the climate we're in, the amount of exercise we get and our individual biochemistry, but on average we need no more than 500 to 1,000 milligrams daily. Most Americans get five or six times this amount every day. This excess can lead to high blood pressure, migraine headaches, abnormal fluid retention or dehydration, and potassium loss. Much of this excess comes from eating processed foods which are loaded with salt and monosodium glutamate (MSG), another form of sodium—yet another reason to eat whole foods!

Eating heavily salted foods is an acquired taste and can be changed. You'll crave salt after exercising and sweating, but under normal circumstances you can easily break a salt habit. If you're eating whole foods, you'll find they're so much tastier you won't need as much salt. Using herbs and spices to make food taste interesting is fun and makes meals creative.

When you do buy processed foods, try to keep the sodium content (listed on all labels) to under 500 milligrams per serving (I consider that high, but I'm being realistic!). Beware, products that are low in sodium are often high in fat or sugar. Your total sodium intake should be no more than 3,000 milligrams per day.

Here are some other places salt is hidden:

- Antacids
- Cough syrups
- Beer
- Baking soda and baking powder
- Laxatives (check the label)
- Home water softeners
- Cured meats such as ham, bologna and hot dogs
- Diet sodas
- Club soda
- Condiments such as pickles, ketchup and mustard
- Soy sauce
- Preservatives such as sodium benzoate and sodium propionate

About half of people with hypertension have excessive sodium. The simplest way to treat this problem is to cut down on salt intake. Some of the drugs doctors prescribe to lower blood pressure are diuretics that cause the body to lose salt, but these have many side effects. It's much healthier to first try lowering blood pressure naturally with diet, exercise and supplements.

CHAPTER 10

Keep Your Fibrinogen Low

You may not have heard a lot about fibrinogen as a risk for heart disease, but its presence is a key factor. Fibrinogen is a protein substance found in blood that plays an important role in blood clotting. In effect, it makes the blood sticky or gummy, but too much makes the blood too sticky.

Fibrinogen is an important substance in the body, being the precursor of fibrin, a non-dissolving protein that plays a major role in the ability of blood to clot. As with so many substances in our body, having enough fibrinogen is essential to good health, but too much is not healthy.

In nearly every study done on heart disease, high levels

of fibrinogen in the blood were found to be directly related to coronary artery disease, probably by interfering with blood flow. Excess fibrinogen is also related to atrial fibrillation, strokes, intermittent claudication (pain in the legs when walking) and high blood pressure. Reducing fibrinogen levels may be your single best protection against having a stroke.

All of the factors that contribute to high fibrinogen, and all the solutions for lowering it, are covered in other chapters in more detail. In other words, most of the factors that raise or lower fibrinogen are the same ones that raise or lower other risk factors for heart disease.

Although researchers don't yet know exactly how fibrinogen works, we do have a pretty good idea of what makes it go up. Women tend to have higher fibrinogen levels, probably because they have more estrogen, which raises it.

WHAT MAKES FIBRINOGEN LEVELS RISE

Psychological and mental stress can increase fibrinogen levels.

High blood sugar raises fibrinogen levels.

Very high LDL cholesterol levels will raise fibrinogen levels.

Estrogen, which is found in birth control pills and in hormone replacement therapy, raises fibrinogen levels, which makes it ironic that the pharmaceutical industry is making claims that estrogen prevents heart disease. It may slightly lower your risk of dying from a heart attack, but it raises your risk of dying from a stroke and from cancer. (More about that in the chapter on hormone replacement therapy.)

Smoking has a direct effect on raising fibrinogen levels.

Obesity signficantly raises fibrinogen levels.

What Lowers Fibrinogen Levels?

Exercise is the single biggest factor in lowering fibrinogen levels.

A glass of wine with dinner may slightly lower fibrinogen levels.

Fish oil supplementation may lower fibrinogen levels.

Eating plenty of garlic lowers fibrinogen.

Olive oil lowers fibrinogen.

Vitamin E lowers fibrinogen.

A vegetarian diet lowers fibrinogen.

A double-blind placebo study of fibrinogen levels in women found that those whose diet was supplemented with fish oil or olive oil had significantly lower levels of fibrinogen, while those on a placebo did not change. Population studies suggest that the risk of having a stroke is two to four times higher in people with high fibrinogen levels.

CHAPTER 11

Keep Your Homocysteine Low with Folic Acid and Other B Vitamins

In the past few years it has been very well scientifically documented that high levels of homocysteine, a byproduct of metabolism of the amino acid methionine, is an important risk factor in heart disease and strokes associated with narrowed blood vessels. In fact, I believe high homocysteine levels will turn out to be a much more accurate marker of heart disease risk than cholesterol or blood pressure.

Researchers currently believe that excess homocysteine damages blood vessels, so it may turn out to be a primary cause of heart disease and not just an indicator. The solution to keeping homocysteine levels low is straightforward for most people. To be neutralized in the body, homocysteine needs B vitamins and hydrochloric acid. A deficiency of any of these can raise homocysteine levels, producing hyperhomocysteinemia, a name I predict you'll be hearing a lot in the next decade or so.

Let's hope it won't be ten or twenty years before mainstream medicine begins admitting that high homocysteine levels are an important risk factor for heart disease. But my guess is that most people will never hear about it because the treatment is so simple and inexpensive. No pharmaceutical company will make excessive profits from this natural treatment!

THE HIDDEN RISK FACTOR

Meanwhile, more than 20 studies involving over 2,000 patients have shown that homocysteine levels are significantly higher in people who have coronary artery disease and strokes. In fact, some researchers speculate that high levels of homocysteine may account for the 30 to 40 percent of people who have heart disease without exhibiting any of the other known risk factors such as high cholesterol, high blood pressure and obesity.

Homocysteine is an amino acid meant to exist only temporarily in the body as a by-product of methionine (another amino acid) metabolism. In a healthy body it's quickly transformed into harmless substances. If you have a deficiency of certain B vitamins, or a genetic predisposition that interferes with the metabolism of homocysteine, the levels of it in your blood will rise, and so will your risk of heart disease and stroke. According to Dr. Mason of Tufts University School of Medicine in Boston, if your homocysteine levels are just 20 percent above normal, your risk of cardiovascular disease is significantly increased. If your doctor wants to measure your homocysteine levels, a normal homocysteine level is about 12 micromols per liter (μmol/L), and cardiovascular risk increases at about 14 to 16 μmol/L.

Scientists know that homocysteine damages arteries, but haven't been able to precisely pin down how. The best evidence suggests that it causes certain kinds of arterial cells called endothelial cells to fall apart. This is the type of damage that attracts cholesterol to the artery walls in an attempt to patch things up. But the "bad" cholesterol accumulates and eventually clogs up the arteries. Antioxidants will help significantly in reducing the amount of "bad" cholesterol in the blood, but if homocysteine levels remain high, the damage to arterial walls will continue.

A large Canadian study evaluated homocysteine levels

in 584 healthy people, and compared them with 150 people with coronary artery disease. Their levels of vitamin B12, B6, pyridoxal phosphate and folic acid were also evaluated. The results clearly showed that the higher the homocysteine, the lower the levels of folic acid, B12 and pyridoxal phosphate (a form of vitamin B6) levels. Those with low levels of these B vitamins and high homocysteine had a higher risk of heart disease.

HOW TO REDUCE HOMOCYSTEINE LEVELS

Some drugs can cause high homocysteine levels, particularly those that interfere with folic acid. These include methotrexate, an immunosuppressive drug given to cancer, rheumatoid arthritis and psoriasis patients; the anticonvulsant drugs phenytoin (Dilantin) and carbamazepine (Tegretol, Epitol); and the bile acid sequestrants for lowering cholesterol levels, cholestipol (Colestid) and cholestyramine (Questran). It's ironic that these cholesterol-lowering drugs, given to reduce heart disease, may actually cause it by raising homocysteine levels!

Other research has shown that homocysteine levels rise when daily folic acid intake is 200 micrograms per day or less. This is a typical example of how inadequate the official RDA (Recommended Dietary Allowance) amounts are, because the current RDA for folate is 200 mcg.

Fortunately, for nearly everyone, homocysteine can be easily and inexpensively lowered by taking some B vitamins. If you're taking a daily multi-vitamin that includes 400 mcg of folic acid, 50 mg of vitamin B6 and 1,000 mcg of vitamin B12, you should be covered. If your homocysteine levels are high, you should be getting an additional 200 mg daily of vitamin B6 (pyridoxine), and 1-4 mg of folic acid daily until your homocysteine levels are back to normal.

Since a deficiency of vitamin B12 can also indirectly

raise homocysteine levels, and since a high intake of folic acid can mask a vitamin B12 deficiency, I suggest you also make sure your intake of vitamin B12 is at least 1,000 mcg per day. Vitamin B12 is best taken sublingually (under the tongue), in a nasal gel or spray, or as an injection.

If you're having trouble with digestion you may want to take a liquid B complex that's easier for your body to absorb.

Adding betaine to your supplements, in the form of betaine hydrochloride, can also aid in lowering homocysteine levels when combined with the B vitamins. Any brand of betaine hydrochloride will be fine—check your health food store and follow the directions on the label.

CHAPTER 12

Magnesium Is Your Most Important Heart Mineral

Magnesium is a mineral found in our cells and bones, and is vital to nearly every major biologic process in the body. It helps maintain fluid and electrical balance in our cells, and is involved with sending messages through the nerves, relaxing smooth muscles and maintaining the integrity of our blood vessels. Magnesium also regulates how we absorb and use calcium and is critical to more than 300 enzyme reactions involved in energy metabolism. This means it is also involved in regulating how the body uses nutrients and other substances such as hormones. For example, both vitamin B6 and vitamin E need magnesium in order to work properly. This important mineral is also part of the process used to break down and absorb proteins.

A deficiency of magnesium can result in a calcium deficiency, especially in the bones. When the calcium is directed away from the bones and into the soft tissue because of a magnesium deficiency, it can cause arthritis symptoms.

A combination of magnesium and vitamin B6 (pyridoxine) has been shown to reduce kidney stones. (The dose used in the study was 300 mg magnesium and 30 mg vitamin B6.) It's also helpful in preventing preeclampsia and eclampsia (toxemia of pregnancy that can include headaches, high blood pressure, nausea and water retention), and some studies even indicate it can help prevent pre-term birth. In some women with PMS, magnesium supplementation can help reduce the symptoms. A magnesium deficiency has also been implicated in migraines. In some studies, up to 80 percent of the people with migraines found relief when they took magnesium supplements. Magnesium has also been found to be useful in treating asthma, anxiety, and can significantly help people with chronic lung disease.

MAGNESIUM AND THE HEALTHY HEART

On top of all these other functions, magnesium plays a central role in maintaining a healthy cardiovascular system. In 1978 it was discovered that in areas where magnesium levels in drinking water were low, the rate of death from heart disease was higher.

Because of magnesium's important role in muscle contraction and cell integrity, a deficiency can negatively affect heart function. Several recent studies have shown that when people come into an emergency room with a heart attack, if they are given intravenous magnesium right away, their chances of survival go way up, and if they continue to receive it their survival rate continues to improve.

A Japanese study published in the *American Journal of Cardiology* found that magnesium deficiency may play a role in coronary artery spasms and in ischemic heart disease, where oxygen is not being delivered to the cells due to a constriction of the blood vessels. Since magnesium is involved in relaxation of the smooth muscles, it can help with almost any kind of spasm, including those of the heart. I believe that a great deal of angina pain could be relieved simply by bringing magnesium levels up to normal.

A magnesium deficiency can lead to irregular heartbeats (arrhythmias). If you're on digitalis for heart disease, the medication can be toxic if you are deficient in potassium or magnesium. Magnesium helps prevent "sticky" blood, and dilates the blood vessels.

A Japanese study found that patients with low HDL (good) cholesterol had low magnesium levels, and that when they took magnesium supplements their HDL levels increased. In addition, animal studies have shown that when magnesium is deficient, the amount of oxidized LDL cholesterol increases, with a corresponding increase in arterial damage.

There have been at least 28 independent studies showing that patients with hypertension (high blood pressure) have a magnesium deficiency. On the average, patients with long-term essential high blood pressure have at least 15 percent below normal magnesium levels.

WHAT DEPLETES MAGNESIUM?

A large study by the U.S. Department of Agriculture found that only 25 percent of 37,785 individuals had magnesium intakes at or greater than the recommended daily allowance. In fact, dietary magnesium intake is only a fraction of the RDA, which is only a measure of what you need to avoid being ill, not what you need to be healthy and energetic. Magnesium imbalances are common in hospitalized patients, with magnesium deficiency occurring in 20 percent to 65 percent of critically ill patients.

Magnesium can be depleted by stress, excessive alcohol, sugar, diabetes, kidney disease, chronic diarrhea, not enough protein in the diet, too much protein in the diet, and thyroid disorders. It's well known that alcoholics are at greater risk for cardiovascular disease and osteoporosis, and this is thought to be caused by the depletion effect excess alcohol has on magnesium.

HOW TO KEEP YOUR MAGNESIUM LEVELS HIGH

Good food sources of magnesium include whole grains (especially oats, brown rice, millet, buckwheat and wheat), legumes (lentils, split peas and beans), bran, almonds, peanuts, and broccoli. Chocolate contains large amounts of magnesium, and a craving for chocolate may be an indicator of a magnesium deficiency.

Magnesium by itself can cause diarrhea, so be sure to take it in a multivitamin, in combination with calcium, and in the form of magnesium glycinate, magnesium citrate or magnesium aspartate.

Most Americans are deficient in magnesium, which is why I recommend you take 300 to 400 mg daily as a supplement. Vegetarians usually have very good magnesium levels—yet another good reason to eat lots of whole grains, fresh fruits and vegetables.

If a health professional wants to test your magnesium levels for some reason, please be aware that since magnesium is found in the highest quantities inside the cells, a blood serum test is not a good indicator of magnesium levels. Have them measure your red blood cell magnesium instead.

CHAPTER 13

Keep Your Antioxidant Status High

Antioxidants come in many forms, from teas and herbal tinctures to foods and vitamins. Their marvelous power gives a shielding, protective effect against heart disease. To learn more about the best-known antioxidants, vitamins C and E, turn to the chapters covering their important individual roles against heart disease. In this chapter I want to tell you about some other important antioxidants that will protect you against heart disease.

ANTIOXIDANTS LOWER YOUR RISK OF HEART DISEASE

Antioxidants score very high as health-promoting factors in population studies reviewing diet, cholesterol levels and rates of heart disease. For example, the *European*

Journal of Clinical Nutrition reported that some Europeans consume more saturated fat than Americans, yet suffer less heart disease. Part of the key is now thought to be the high level of antioxidants in their diet, mainly from plentiful fruits and vegetables. (Although red wine also provides antioxidants, its benefits have been shown only to apply with moderate intake.)

Japan has the second lowest rate of heart disease in the world for women and the lowest rate for men. The Japanese diet, as well as being high in vegetables and fiber and low in fat, is specifically high in antioxidant-rich foods such as soy and green tea. Where high levels of antioxidants are consumed, rates of heart disease are lower.

THE NATURAL POWER OF ANTIOXIDANTS

When a squirt of lemon juice helps food stay fresh, it is working as an antioxidant, protecting against the harmful effects of oxygen. Oxygen harmful? Well, we've all seen rust and tasted rancid oil. Although essential for life, oxygen can also work against it. Unstable oxygen molecules do the damage when their basic paired units, electrons, lose their partners. If an oxygen molecule loses an electron, it stabilizes itself by grabbing another from any body substance or tissue nearby, causing that molecule in turn to become unstable. Every molecule robbed of an electron becomes destabilized itself, and if antioxidants aren't present a chain reaction can take place, creating damage to tissues. This process is called oxidation and is what antioxidants prevent. Unstable oxygen molecules are called free radicals.

Antioxidants work by preventing oxidants from forming, or by putting the brakes on free radical chain reactions. They form part of a well-balanced system that also repairs oxidation damage and neutralizes toxins.

Oxidants are a natural result of the production of energy in our tissues, and they do serve many useful purposes in the body. However, a normally healthy body is designed to keep free radicals in check or directed only where they are useful, such as attacking invading bacteria. Out-of-control oxidation is a causative factor in much illness, including heart disease and strokes. Today's polluted world means our bodies have to cope with far higher levels of free radicals than ever before. Free radical culprits include smog, cigarette smoke, pesticides and food additives. The average American doesn't eat nearly enough antioxidant-rich fresh fruits and vegetables to counteract these environmental toxins. Our bodies are in double oxidant jeopardy, which makes taking antioxidant supplements an important part of preventing heart disease.

ANTIOXIDANTS AND THE CHOLESTEROL CONNECTION

Cholesterol is essential for the formation of many important substances in the body, including steroid hormones. High levels of "good" HDL cholesterol actually help to prevent heart disease. It is elevated levels of "bad" LDL cholesterol that are known to contribute to heart disease. The trouble comes from oxidized LDL cholesterol. Destabilized, it damages blood vessel walls, beginning the build-up of artery-blocking plaque.

Unlike drugs, which may lower "bad" cholesterol levels, but do not tackle the underlying cause, antioxidants work directly against the oxidation of LDL cholesterol. In fact, low levels of antioxidants in the body could be said to be one of the causes of heart disease, since low antioxidants mean high oxidized LDL cholesterol which, in turn, can lead to cardiovascular problems, stroke and heart attack.

One of the many studies showing that antioxidants reduce LDL cholesterol was performed by the NIH (National Institutes of Health). An antioxidant combination of 30 mg of beta-carotene, 800 IU of vitamin E and 1000 mg of vitamin C was taken by 19 middle-aged people with high LDL levels. After one month, the rate of oxidation was decreased by 26 percent and the onset of oxidation had been delayed significantly.

HEART DISEASE AND BETA-CAROTENE

In 1993, researchers reviewing the diets of 87,000 nurses reported an interesting connection between eating carrots or spinach and the risk of stroke. A 68 percent lower risk of stroke was found in nurses eating five or more servings of carrots a week than in those eating one or less a month. Eating spinach each day produced a 43 percent lower risk than for women consuming less. Both vegetables are rich in beta-carotene.

In the Physicians' Health Study a group of 333 doctors with angina pectoris and coronary revascularization, beta-carotene supplementation at 50 mg on alternate days was shown to produce a remarkable 44 percent drop in all major coronary events including death and a 49 percent fall in cardiovascular problems, including stroke and death.

A report from The Netherlands described how a study of 674 heart attack patients supported the theory that beta-carotene may protect against heart attacks by protecting polyunsaturated fatty acids from oxidation.

GETTING THE BETA-CAROTENE YOU NEED

Taking a multivitamin and eating a lot of fresh fruits and vegetables may provide enough beta-carotene. But if there's any doubt, a 10,000 to 25,000 IU daily supplement is recommended. Beta-carotene is best taken with meals, giving most benefit when it is consumed with fatty foods.

HEART DISEASE AND GINKGO BILOBA

Ginkgo biloba extract is made from the tree of the same name. It is particularly rich in antioxidant substances which act synergistically. One of its properties leads to improvement in circulation to the heart. As might be expected, it also reduces oxidized LDL cholesterol levels and lowers LDL cholesterol generally. In addition, it raises "good" HDL cholesterol, and lowers blood fat levels.

THE BEST WAY TO TAKE GINKGO BILOBA

Ginkgo biloba takes time to produce its effects and should be taken in repeated doses for a fairly long period of time. Ginkgo biloba extract (GBE) with at least 24 percent ginkgoflavoglycosides, is the best form to take. Standardized, semi-purified and concentrated, GBE provides consistent levels of its most active compounds. Take the recommended dosage on the package up to 3 or 4 times a day.

HEART DISEASE AND GLUTATHIONE

Glutathione (GSH) is one of the most universal and important antioxidants, particularly renowned for its detoxification properties. As a protein made up of three amino acids, cysteine, glycine and glutamic acid, GSH is called a tripeptide. It is found in the cells of almost all living organisms and represents the frontline of your body's antioxidant defenses. In fact, we could not survive without it.

GSH catches free radicals before they start chain reactions. Then it neutralizes them, and hands them on to compounds such as vitamin E before starting the cycle again. GSH also binds to toxic substances in the liver, aiding their excretion, and neutralizes free radicals threatening red blood cells. As a partner with selenium, glutathione protects the blood, the heart and other or gans as a coenzyme, changing toxic oxidants into more manageable forms.

Higher cholesterol, higher body weight and a 24 per cent higher rate of illness and death were all linked to low levels of GSH in one study of elderly people in England.

HOW TO KEEP YOUR GLUTATHIONE LEVEL HIGH

When you have a good supply of glutathione's three amino acid components, GSH is constantly renewable extremely abundant and highly active in your body. If you have high LDL cholesterol levels or are otherwise a risk of heart disease, it is worth trying to raise your GSH levels. Of the three, cysteine is the amino acid more liable to run short, and can be taken as the supplement NAC (N-acetyl cysteine). Be sure to follow label recommendations and do not overdose, as the body chemistry in this area is in delicate balance. Foods high in cysteine include wheat germ, red meat, yogurt, onions and garlic

Overexposure to drugs which are hard on the liver such as aspirin and Tylenol, and an overload of rancid oils, can deplete GSH levels. Aging also causes GSH levels to fall. Keep up your levels of selenium and vitamins C and E to ensure that GSH works efficiently in the body with these nutrient partners.

HEART DISEASE AND GREEN TEA

Green tea is a polyphenol, an aromatic, organic compound that acts as a potent antioxidant in the body. Like others in this family it prevents the oxidation of LDL cholesterol, lowers cholesterol, raises "good" HDL levels and lowers triglyceride levels. It also reduces blood coagulation and prevents the clumping of red blood cells, both good steps for the prevention of heart disease.

Studies in Japan have shown that green tea even out-erforms synthetic vitamin E, vitamin C, a synthetic anti-xidant called BHT and glutathione when it comes to he prevention of oxidation in fatty substances.

HEART DISEASE AND PCOs

COs are procyanidolic oligomers which are bioflavo-oids found in grapeseed, lemon tree bark, peanuts, ranberries and citrus peels. Known to improve circula-on, PCOs strengthen blood vessel walls and prevent the lumping of bood clotting substances, protecting against troke. These properties come on top of PCOs' very trong antioxidant powers that preempt LDL oxidation.

TAKING PCO SUPPLEMENTS

'o address high cholesterol with PCOs, 150 to 300 mg er day is recommended. Otherwise, 50 mg of PCOs aily makes a good supplement if you're over 50. Many tudies have shown that PCO extract from grapeseed is ne of the most powerful antioxidants known. It also ncreases the performance of other antioxidants.

The best grapeseed extract is packaged with "phyto-omes," a process in which the molecules are combined ith a natural component of lecithin. This combination ncreases the absorption and effectiveness of the PCO in our body.

MAKING YOUR DIET ANTIOXIDANT-RICH

our main food sources of antioxidants are fresh fruits nd vegetables. Top scorers are: cabbage, cauliflower and roccoli; spinach and kale and other dark green, leafy egetables; carrots, sweet potatoes and other "yellow" egetables; garlic and onions.

Remember, some antioxidants such as vitamin C are

lost when you boil vegetables. Eat vegetables steamed o
raw if you don't want to see your heart protection g
down the drain!

CHAPTER 14

Vitamin E Is Your Most Important Heart Vitamin

Vitamin E is your greatest ally and protector when
comes to vitamins and heart health, and yet most peop
are deficient in vitamin E. In one study, the vitamin
intake of elderly, affluent Americans was less than thre
quarters of the RDA.

A World Health Organization (WHO) review of Eur
pean populations, nutrient levels and health showed th
those with higher levels of vitamin E had a lower rate
coronary artery disease. The same result held, eve
where saturated fat intakes were high, in non-Europe:
and European countries.

Impressive results were shown in two major Harva
University studies of health professionals. A survey
over 39,000 male professionals showed that they enjoye
a 37 percent lower risk of coronary artery disease whe
they took 100 IU or more of vitamin E daily. The Nurse

Health Study of 87,000 women showed a 40 percent lower risk of heart disease for women on the same dose of vitamin E.

A European population study looked at 100 apparently healthy men aged 40 to 49 years old. Blood levels of vitamin E were found to be the most important risk factor for heart disease, even beyond smoking. Levels of vitamins E and A in the blood were so significant that researchers could use them with 73 percent accuracy to predict which of the men studied would die from a heart attack.

VITAMIN E KEEPS BLOOD VESSELS FREE ...

Vitamin E is the oldest recognized biological antioxidant. Animal and human studies done at the University of Texas Southwestern Medical Center have shown that supplementation with vitamin E reduces the extent of "bad" LDL cholesterol oxidation. Studies by Japanese scientists have also shown that vitamin E reduces levels of oxidized fats in the bloodstream. Vitamin E also works closely with glutathione, an antioxidant enzyme that is particularly important to the layer of cells which line the heart, blood and lymph vessels.

Swedish researchers working with rabbits and high cholesterol concluded that vitamin E supplementation halted and in some cases even reversed arterial damage caused by oxidation.

... AND FLOWING

Several studies show that vitamin E inhibits the release of clotting agents in the bloodstream which cause blood to clump and clot, increasing the risk of stroke. A report in the *American Journal of Clinical Nutrition* on vascular disease of the legs, which often occurs with heart disease, described how patients treated with vitamin E enjoyed increased blood flow, less painful walking and far fewer amputations. Another study looked at 1,476 patients with general atherosclerosis who had taken supplemental vitamin E for ten years. The patients' ten-year survival rate was higher than for any patients in similar studies who had not been treated with vitamin E.

There is evidence, too, that vitamin E can dissolve clots, helps the heart pump more efficiently, naturally makes arteries widen and increases the oxygen available in the blood.

How to Get the Vitamin E You Need

Vitamin E is a fat-soluble oil found in many foods, including unrefined vegetable oils, whole grains, butter, organ meats, eggs, a variety of nuts, sunflower seeds, fruit, soybeans and dark green leafy vegetables.

I recommend that you take vitamin E either mixed as tocopherols or d-alpha tocopherol. I do not recommend the synthetic form of vitamin E, called dl-alpha tocopherol.

Although vitamin E is very safe even at high doses, 400 IU to 800 IU (dry form) daily should be an adequate dose for adults. The dry form is recommended for anyone sensitive to oils or with problems absorbing nutrients (if you're over the age of 65 you probably fall into the latter category). Vitamin E works well taken with its partners in the body, the nutrients vitamin C, beta-carotene and other flavonoids, and selenium.

CHAPTER 15

Vitamin C Makes Everything Work Better

It's now well established that vitamin C, which is ascorbic acid, has a preventive and therapeutic effect against infectious diseases like the common cold. It is, in fact, important for a wide range of bodily functions from the production of antistress hormones to the healing of wounds. An increasing number of studies show that vitamin C is also highly valuable as protection against heart disease.

Several population studies single out vitamin C intake as a major factor protecting against heart disease. Over 40 years ago, a California study concluded that vitamin C was the most important of 25 factors in preventing death—the most usual cause of which was heart disease. Another study of a large population in England found vitamin C to give the greatest protective effect against ischemic heart disease caused by a narrowing and constriction of the blood vessels.

"C" FOR CHOLESTEROL CONTROL

Vitamin C is useful against that known heart disease villain, "bad" LDL cholesterol. It's important to remember that most of our cholesterol is made within our bodies, and studies show that high-cholesterol foods do not cause significant changes in blood cholesterol. LDL cholesterol becomes harmful when it is oxidized by free radicals. Vitamin C works directly against internally generated oxidized LDL. As early as 1947, a study in Russia showed vitamin C could bring down high cholesterol levels. Many studies since then have confirmed this result.

One of the ways the body regulates cholesterol is by converting it into bile acids which are excreted into the intestines. When the body needs more cholesterol, it will reabsorb some of the bile acids and pull out the cholesterol. Two good studies have shown that the rate at which cholesterol is removed from the blood by being converted into bile acids is increased by a high intake of vitamin C. In addition, vitamin C can act as a laxative, speeding up the removal of bile acids from the bowel. This, of course, means less bile acids get converted back into cholesterol.

A German study gave patients with high cholesterol levels one gram of vitamin C per day for three months. The patients saw their cholesterol levels drop by an average of 10 percent. Another German study looked at patients with extremely high cholesterol levels, and found an even greater average drop of 18 percent in cholesterol levels when the patients were given three grams of vitamin C for just three weeks.

Vitamin C produces little change in people with normal cholesterol levels. One researcher studied 280 men and women with a range of low to high cholesterol levels. Given 300 to 1000 mg of vitamin C, average cholesterol levels stayed the same in people with normal cholesterol, and decreased by 10 to 20 percent for those with high cholesterol.

Additional evidence of vitamin C's beneficial role in cholesterol regulation comes from recent studies showing that vitamin C not only lowers levels of "bad" LDL cholesterol, but also raises "good" HDL levels.

Vitamin C and Cardiovascular Disease

Vitamin C is indirectly beneficial to the heart through its partnership with vitamin E. Vitamin E is an antioxidant which helps prevent the oxidation of unsaturated fatty acids and LDL cholesterol. Vitamin C is also an antioxidant, but has a special role in restoring "spent" vitamin E.

Thrombosis or blood clotting in the coronary arteries is a major cause of heart attacks. The root cause is the body's blood clotting system going seriously awry. Studies show that a deficiency of vitamin C often lies behind this.

It's known that people with coronary artery disease have lower levels of vitamin C than healthy people. In one study of postsurgical patients, the number of blood clots developed in patients given one gram of vitamin C daily was significantly lower than that in patients who did not receive the supplement. The research shows the chemistry of vitamin C both boosts clot-dissolving activity and inhibits the clumping of cells that leads to clots. These actions make it a valuable heart disease preventive.

Increase Vitamin C, Decrease Blood Pressure

As well as helping to prevent blood clotting, studies show that a diet high in vitamin C helps keep blood pressure down. Research on elderly people performed at the U.S. Department of Agriculture's Human Nutrition Research Center on Aging showed that taking the amount of vitamin C in four oranges a day kept blood pressure four times lower than did eating the vitamin C in one orange.

Research shows that low levels of vitamin C raise both systolic and diastolic blood pressure readings. It's clear that a diet rich in vitamin C is a simple way to help treat high blood pressure, a condition which plagues over 60 million Americans and is intimately linked to heart attacks and strokes.

How to Boost Your Vitamin C

Statistics show that vitamin C is the most widely taken dietary supplement. It cannot be made in the body and must come from food or supplements. There is evidence that taking flavonoids with vitamin C raises its concentrations in some tissues and helps to trigger some of its effects.

Because some vitamin C is lost through excretion, it's best taken in a dose divided throughout the day. Recommended levels vary, but 500 mg twice daily should be sufficient for adults and children over ten. Illness, stress, smoking and injury all increase the need for vitamin C. Megadoses of vitamin C can wash out B12 and folic acid, so increase your B vitamins if you're taking a lot of vitamin C.

Of course, supplementation is no substitute for a diet naturally rich in vitamin C. Fresh fruits (especially citrus) and vegetables are the best source. Raw is best, as cooking destroys vitamin C. Include vitamin C in a low-fat, low-sugar, high-fiber diet with lots of fish and little meat, and your heart will be well protected.

CHAPTER 16

Use My Two Favorite Heart Strengtheners, CoQ10 and Hawthorn Berries

One of the best-kept secrets around is the well-proven ability of a nutrient called coenzyme Q10 (CoQ10) to protect and strengthen the heart, to lower blood pressure, to strengthen the immune system, and as an added bonus, to cure gum disease. It also happens to be extremely safe and nontoxic.

CoQ10 is a vital enzyme, or catalyst to the production of energy in our cells. Without it, our cells simply won't work. Its chemical name is *ubiquinone*—it is ubiquitous, or everywhere, where there is life. Its levels in the human body are highest in the heart and liver. When we are ill or stressed, and as we age, our bodies are less able to produce CoQ10.

According to a study done by CoQ10 expert Karl Folkers, published in the *International Journal of Vitamin and Nutrition Research,* patients with a variety of cardiac disorders consistently demonstrate a blood deficiency of CoQ10. A double-blind Japanese study with 100 patients who had cardiac failure showed that as little as 30 mg per day of CoQ10 for two to four weeks produced a measurable improvement in symptoms. Many older people whose heart function has degenerated and who try CoQ10 report an almost immediate boost in their energy levels.

People who suffer from angina report that the pain disappears and they can do some exercise. In a double-blind placebo study using CoQ10 and other drugs traditionally used to treat angina, it was found that CoQ10 was far more effective in reducing or eliminating angina pain than any of the other medications. Other studies have shown that people on heart medications can greatly reduce their dosage of medicine if it is combined with CoQ10.

I know you're asking the question, "If this stuff is so good, why isn't it being prescribed for everyone who has heart disease?" Like so many of the heart helpers in this book, CoQ10 is a natural substance, so it can't be patented. Therefore the drug companies can't have exclusive use of it or charge high prices for it, so they have no interest in selling it, no reason to promote it, and in fact have every reason to wish it would go away. There are literally volumes of good research done on CoQ10, much of it sponsored by the government.

HOW TO TAKE COQ10

CoQ10 should come as a powder in a capsule and be a deep yellow color. It it's not, or if it's cut with fillers, find a brand that's pure and the right color. Also be sure that the product says "coenzyme Q10" or "CoQ10." Variations of it will not be as effective. The purity and quality of CoQ10 do vary, and since it's not a cheap supplement, it pays to get a high-quality brand. Most CoQ10 comes in 30 mg capsules and costs about $16 for 100 capsules. You can take one 30 mg capsule up to three times a day with meals.

If you want to know more about CoQ10, get a paperback book called *The Miracle Nutrient: Coenzyme Q10,* by Emile G. Bliznakov, M.D. and Gerald L. Hunt.

HAWTHORN BERRIES

Hawthorn berries (*Crataegus oxyacantha*) have been used as heart tonic for centuries and are widely used in Europe s a heart medicine for angina and for lowering blood ressure. They are rich in bioflavonoids, which help rengthen the blood vessels. They are also a vasodilator, which increases the flow of blood and oxygen to the heart, owers blood pressure and strengthens the heart muscle.

Hawthorn berries work gradually, and you may not otice a difference for a month or so. You can find haw- horn berries in capsule or tincture forms. Because the mounts vary widely, follow directions for use on the ottle. Some of the tinctures can be very powerful, so it s very important, if you're already on heart medicine, hat you work with your physician. However, in and of hemselves, hawthorn berries are very nontoxic and safe.

CHAPTER 17

f You Need Hormones, Take the Natural Ones

That estrogen protects against heart disease has become n accepted "fact" in mainstream medicine, but in real- ty there is little evidence to support this claim. The supposed benefits of estrogen are much less well established than drug company advertising would have you believe, but the increased risk of cancer and stroke are very well established.

We do know that estrogen can improve lipid profiles slightly (raise HDL cholesterol and lower LDL cholesterol), but it's a big leap to say that therefore it must also protect against dying from heart disease, especially considering that estrogen raises fibrinogen levels, a significant risk factor for heart disease.

The mainstay of the claim that estrogen will prevent heart disease is the famous Harvard Nurses' Study. But the information regarding estrogen in this study is seriously flawed. First of all, two very unequal groups of women were compared. Doctors do not (or should not) prescribe estrogen to women who are obese, diabetic, have kidney or liver disease, are at a risk for cancer or stroke, or smoke cigarettes. Therefore, the women who took estrogen were, by elimination, a healthier group to begin with, and less likely to have heart disease with or without the hormone replacement therapy. (Other studies also show that women who use hormone replacement therapy are more likely to be better educated and healthier.) To the best of my knowledge, there are no other studies showing that estrogen or hormone replacement therapy of any kind truly reduces the risk of dying from heart disease.

Furthermore, the women in this study who took estrogen had a much higher risk of stroke, even though they were a healthier group.

The *New England Journal of Medicine* published a study by the highly respected Harvard researcher Dr. Graham Colditz, showing that women who use estrogen for more than a few years have a 46 percent higher risk of breast cancer. Colditz is one of the primary authorities on the link between estrogen and breast cancer, and his results came from more than 121,700 women tracked for 2 ears in the Harvard Nurses' Study. It is also well established that estrogen causes ovarian cancer.

In addition to an increased risk of stroke, breast cancer, and ovarian cancer, estrogen causes weight gain, bloating, headaches, irritability, depression, tender breasts, fatigue, thinning of scalp hair, foggy thinking, and decreased libido. Why would anyone want to subject themselves to that?

GETTING WHAT YOU REALLY NEED AT MENOPAUSE

Somehow mainstream medicine has forgotten about the important role the hormone progesterone plays in a woman's hormonal cycles. A woman's level of progesterone actually drops much more dramatically at menopause than estrogen levels do, and this accounts for more of the menopausal symptoms than a drop in estrogen does.

Progesterone is actually confused, even by otherwise competent doctors, with the synthetic progestins found in birth control pills and hormone replacement therapy (Provera, for example), but one is a safe, natural hormone and the other is a dangerous synthetic drug. They are most emphatically not the same.

Progesterone has no known side effects other than some sleepiness at very high doses, but the progestins have a long list of negative side effects. For example, the progestins can cause miscarriage and fetal malformation, but progesterone is essential for a successful pregnancy. This alone should be a major clue to physicians and their patients that these two substances are very different. The progestins also cause bloating, headaches, weight gain, breast tenderness, depression, migraines, asthma, breakthrough bleeding, liver damage, decreased glucose tolerance, excess hair growth, and an increased risk of stroke. Makes you wonder why it's allowed on the market, doesn't it?

All of the maladies for which doctors are prescribing estrogen can be prevented and reversed with diet and lifestyle changes and, when necessary, with some natural progesterone cream. (Please do not confuse natural progesterone cream, which is often identified on the label as "wild yam extract" with another "wild yam extract" substance called diosgenin. Some manufacturers are claiming that diosgenin becomes progesterone in the body, and are selling it as progesterone. Diosgenin is no progesterone, and there is no evidence whatsoever that it becomes progesterone in the body. Diosgenin is used to make natural progesterone in the laboratory, but no in the body!)

Progesterone does not raise fibrinogen levels, and high levels of it in the body are actually associated with a reduced risk of breast cancer. It will also raise HDL level and lower LDL levels as well or better than estrogen.

It is very well known now that heart disease is one of the most preventable of all chronic diseases with diet and life style changes. Why should a woman increase her risk of breast cancer by 46 percent, her risk of stroke by up to 4 percent and suffer from all the estrogen and progestin side effects, when she can accomplish the same thing naturally and increase her quality of life in every way?

Women who keep their weight within reasonable limits, who keep their fat intake low and their vegetable intake high, and who get some regular exercise, rarely suffer from distressing menopause symptoms. Those who add soy products such as soy milk and tofu to their daily diet are even less likely to complain about menopause symptoms. High soy consumption and low fat consumption are almost certainly the primary reasons that hot flashes and breast cancer are virtually unknown in Japan.

Estrogen's benefits for osteoporosis have also been greatly exaggerated. It will slow bone loss for a few years around the time of menopause, but after that it has no benefit. Women who are at risk for osteoporosis can pre ent it with a combination of diet (not too much protein, a minimum of carbonated beverages, and plenty of fresh vegetables), weight-bearing exercise and some progesterone cream, which has been convincingly shown by Dr. John Lee to stimulate bone growth and reverse osteoporosis.

For a very small percentage of women, diet, exercise and natural progesterone do not relieve them of menopause symptoms such as severe hot flashes and vaginal dryness. If you fall into this category, find a doctor who will give you a small amount of natural estrogen, rather than something like Premarin, which is made from pregnant mares' urine.

If you decide to use natural progesterone, please do so with an experienced health care practitioner and use a brand known to contain actual progesterone.

CHAPTER 18

Get Moving and Shed the Extra Pounds

Our bodies are designed to move. Movement is essential for health, and exercise is simply a way of making sure your body gets the movement it needs. Scientific research has shown us that the internal benefits of exercise include improved circulation, increased oxygen uptake better lymph circulation and therefore better immune functions and elimination of toxins. Digestion and absorption improve, and muscles, joints, tendons and ligaments are all strengthened. Exercise is especially good for the heart but, really, every part of the body benefits

If you've been a couch potato, once you begin exercising you'll soon experience many worthwhile "side effects" of exercise. People who exercise regularly find they have more energy, can relax and unwind more easily and sleep better. Many say their mood brightens, stress tolerance increases, and even their sex life improves! Exercise for a healthy heart and you'll gain much more besides—except weight of course—unless it's muscle weight you're building.

EXERCISE LOWERS RISK FACTORS

You can show the power of a really good laundry detergent by using it on very dirty clothes. Well, the power of exercise is demonstrated when it improves the health of smokers. This was the case in a study from the University of California. A group of 28 healthy female cigarette smokers (averaging 17 cigarettes a day for an average of 20 years) was studied. After exercise, it was found they enjoyed a reduction in risk factors for coronary artery disease and stroke. Levels of harmful agents in the blood came down and oxygen uptake improved. And they didn't have to become fanatics to get these benefits. Any exercise program over two hours per week for longer than six months produced a decreased risk of coronary artery disease.

Further evidence comes from a French study which showed that if physical exercise is sustained it can reduce fibrinogen in the blood and therefore reduce the risk of having a stroke.

EXERCISE AND CHOLESTEROL

Running seven to 14 miles a week can increase your levels of HDL cholesterol. This was shown in a study of 2,906 healthy, nonsmoking males by the Veterans Affairs Medical Center. What's more, ratios of HDL to "bad" LDL cholesterol also improved. Don't overdo it, however. No more heart protection advantage seems to come from running further, but the risk of joint injury goes up.

EXERCISE AND BLOOD PRESSURE

A New Zealand study found that individuals with hypertension who walked briskly for 40 minutes three times a week showed significant reductions in systolic blood pressure. Along similar lines, a Belgian lifestyle research study showed a connection between blood pressure and exercise. As calories were burned up in sports, so blood pressure, and therefore risk of heart disease, went down.

GET THINNER, LIVE LONGER

Men who were thinnest at the beginning of a 27-year study were more than twice as likely to be alive at the end of it. This was the result of a study of 19,297 men by the Harvard School of Public Health. Keep that heart ticking—exercise to lose that excess weight!

GET ON THE MOVE—STARTING NOW!

Research shows most Americans have as much trouble sticking to exercise as they do sticking to a diet! Part of the solution lies in making your life itself a workout that you don't have to think about. Walk the dog. Join your children playing. Walk or bike to work and during your lunch hour. Get busy with chores and kill two birds with one stone. Raking, digging, weeding are all good aerobic movement. Weather bad? Dusting, mopping, sweeping—

add them all to your exercise list. Park a few blocks away, use stairs instead of elevators. Even standing instead of sitting to watch TV is helpful! Add a few on-the-spot stretches, too. Get moving!

In addition to movement as part of life, the trick is to make exercise as much a priority as eating or sleeping, and to make it enjoyable. Plan an exercise schedule and, at least for the first six months, build in support like classes, videos, exercise partners, and weekend recreation.

WALK YOUR HEART TO HEALTH

Simple and easy, one of the best physical workouts is a brisk, daily 30 minute walk. Starting from scratch, three days a week is fine, building up gradually to about two miles in a half hour. Remember, always consult your doctor first if you have a medical condition that might make brisk walking hazardous to your health.

Equipment is minimal and inexpensive: A good pair of walking shoes rather than tennis or running shoes with energy-absorbing soles to lessen the strain on your ankles, knees, hips and back; cotton and Lycra walking socks with reinforced heels and toes, as toes and heels are stressed when you walk quickly.

As you walk, move your arms in time with your pace. You'll find your whole body perspires a little by the end of your walk. Using weights gives the upper body more of a workout and, of course, your heart is an upper body muscle. Start with one-pound hand weights and build up gradually to four or five pounds each over about a year. Aim at a pace around three or four miles per hour, which is a mile every 15 to 20 minutes. An inexpensive pedometer can help you figure out the mileage. As much as possible, gear your walk to a time of day when your energy levels are high, remembering that urban pollution levels are lowest in the morning before rush hour.

Get outdoors with local walking or hiking groups or take designated walking routes in your local shopping malls. Find friends to join you in this very simple way to protect your heart.

MOVE THE EASTERN WAY

Instead of fast, sweaty aerobics, you might prefer to give your heart a workout with the gentler mind-body-spirit approach of the Eastern movement arts of yoga and chi kung (or qi gong). Begin by taking a class. Follow up with books and video tapes if you enjoy them. A number of videos on chi kung, tai'chi (a form of chi kung) and yoga are available from The Sounds True Catalog (1-800-333-9185).

CHAPTER 19

"Life's Too Mysterious, Don't Take It Serious"

Stress is a major contributor to heart disease, and the title of this chapter, which I first saw on a greeting card, sums up a heart-healthy approach to life. I don't mean to suggest that we should shirk personal responsibility, but that we could all benefit from approaching life with a sense of humor, a sense of detached compassion for ourselves or others when we can't change things we don't like, and a sense of possibility for the wonders that each day can bring us. As any healthy 90-year-old will tell you, life's true value is found in time spent with loved ones, helping others, laughter, fun and, for many, a spiritual focus.

HOW THE HEART RESPONDS TO STRESS

Mental and emotional stress cause the body to react as if it's in danger, increasing heart rate and blood pressure, releasing adrenaline that makes us jittery and tense, increasing muscle tension, and shunting blood away from digestion and other organ functions. Constant stress causes wear and tear that sooner or later will show up as illness: heart disease, stroke, headaches, chronic pain, back problems, indigestion and psychological disorders such as anxiety and compulsive behavior.

Recent research has given us even more detail on how stress causes heart disease. When blood pressure rises due to stress, the heart responds by narrowing arteries which can cause them to spasm and increase blood clotting factors. When stress occurs over a long enough period of time, the heart muscle simply begins to wear out, and if nutritional deficiencies are present, such as low B vitamins, antioxidants or magnesium, that will accelerate the chances of having a heart attack or stroke.

There are even prominent researchers who have studied stress and cholesterol levels who believe that stress plays a much greater role in raising cholesterol levels than diet. (Actually, there is very little evidence that high cholesterol foods raise cholesterol levels in the body, but that's another story!)

The evidence that stress plays a major role in heart

disease is so overwhelming that some insurance companies are now paying for their high-risk policy holders to participate in lifestyle programs designed by Dr. Dean Ornish to reverse heart disease. These programs include a low-fat vegetarian diet, participation in a support group, an exercise program and meditation.

THE RELAXATION RESPONSE

When Dr. Herbert Benson published the book *The Relaxation Response* more than 20 years ago, it was part of a revolutionary new concept: that by de-stressing our lives we could be healthier, happier people. This especially applies to heart disease. Since then we've also discovered that having frequent feelings of anger, hostility, powerlessness or loneliness can also contribute significantly to heart disease.

A number of studies have found that people who feel isolated and alone and without a sense of community are as much as twice as likely as the "averagely" sociable to have a heart attack. Even having a pet can alleviate some of these feelings, but volunteering at a local soup kitchen will help even more.

It's also very helpful to learn a relaxation response, such as a form of meditation or a breathing exercise, that you can use when you feel tension arising. As mentioned in the chapter on exercise, yoga and chi kung are Eastern disciplines that incorporate a relaxation response into their practice. In fact, many hospitals now routinely teach yoga or chi kung to their heart attack patients. One study showed that people with high blood pressure who participated in support groups, learned a relaxation response and got some exercise were able to lower their blood pressure significantly enough to reduce their blood pressure medication by 80 percent, and 20 percent of them were able to stop using it altogether.

TRY THESE NUTRITIONAL DE-STRESSORS

Certain nutritional deficiencies can increase your mental and emotional stress levels. These include the B vitamins, which help regulate brain function, and the minerals calcium and magnesium, which play a part in relaxing muscles. For some people, a sublingual B vitamin is just the ticket to an energy boost that can be calming at the same time. If you know you're going to be under a lot of stress, be sure to increase your intake of these supplements.

If you're under stress, please avoid stimulants. Especially avoid drinking too much coffee. More than two or three cups will make you jittery, deplete your adrenal glands, and rob you of needed vitamins and minerals. Also avoid sugar. It can pick up your energy for a short time, but you're likely to feel even lower as little as a half hour later. If you're craving something sweet, try fruit, which contains a lot of sugar, but in a form better tolerated by the body. A banana contains potassium, which will calm you down, natural sugars, which will give you a bit of a lift, and carbohydrates, which will give you long-term energy.

Ginseng tea gives a lift without stressing out the adrenal glands and without a letdown. It actually supports and balances the body. A brisk walk can get your circulatory and lymphatic systems moving, making you more alert.

The bottom line is that it's not healthy to be stressed out all the time, and there are many ways to alleviate and eliminate stress. Start today and your heart will thank you for the rest of your life.

CHAPTER 20

Is Your Heart Drug Doing More Harm Than Good?

As a pharmacist, I'm well versed in just how much damage prescription drugs, and particularly drugs to treat heart disease, can do to people. Over the past few decades it's become clear that prescription drugs are not the magic bullets we thought they would be. It's true that these drugs have saved many lives, but it's also increasingly true that they are taking a great many lives and ruining even more with debilitating side effects.

One quarter of the elderly population, or 6.6 million people, are taking a drug they should never take. Many people are prescribed a drug, then prescribed another one to counter the side effects of the first, and then a third to counter the side effects of the first two. I call this getting on the drug treadmill. People typically get out on the drug treadmill by their doctor in their 60s, and never get off it. The average senior citizen is taking eight different drugs every day!

According to government figures, some 140,000 people die every year from pharmaceutical drugs, and many more are hospitalized. This is absolutely unnecessary. I don't want you to be part of those statistics. I believe that the side effects of prescription drugs cause most symptoms of aging such as fatigue, forgetfulness and impotence. I want you to take as few prescription drugs as possible, and learn to treat risk factors for heart disease

such as high blood pressure and high cholesterol natu
rally. That simply means following the steps I have out
lined in this book.

It's important to make the distinction between a drug
that effectively treats a symptom and a drug that actually
reduces the chance that you'll die from a heart attack.
Most heart disease drugs treat the symptom effectively,
such as lowering blood pressure or cholesterol, but not
the underlying problem, and your risk of dying of heart
disease remains the same. If these drugs were working
such wonders, the United States wouldn't continue to
have the highest rate of death from heart disease in
the world!

You can avoid the vast majority of pharmaceutical
drugs simply by using the information I've given you in
this book. When you do need to treat a cold, allergy,
illness or symptom of aging, you can nearly always use
simple, effective natural remedies and herbs.

If you're not taking any prescription drugs, congratu
late yourself. And if your doctor wants to put you on
one, go on the defensive. Ask some important questions
such as: Exactly what will this drug do? How long will I
need to take it? Are there any safe, effective ways to treat
this problem without drugs? Is this the lowest dose I can
take? What are the side effects?

If you are on a prescription drug, I don't want
you to go off it without consulting your doctor. At
the same time, I encourage you to consider how much
your quality of life will improve if you treat heart dis
ease symptoms with the suggestions I've given you in
this book rather than with drugs that reduce your qual
ity of life with their unpleasant side effects. I realize
it's more difficult to change old habits than to pop a
pill, but the benefit you will receive in a better quality
of life and increased energy will make it well worth
the effort.

TREATING HIGH BLOOD PRESSURE AND CHOLESTEROL

Taking medication to lower blood pressure or cholesterol should not have to be a fact of life for so many Americans. The truth is that these drugs don't work very well to lower your risk of dying from heart disease, and most of them will make you feel awful. Diuretics used to lower blood pressure can starve your body of minerals important to your heart function such as magnesium, and actually raise your risk of disease. Drugs that lower cholesterol can make you feel tired and impotent, and increase your risk of dying in an accident or committing suicide.

It's important to always begin treating mild to moderate high blood pressure and high LDL cholesterol with nondrug methods. The biggest risk factors for both high blood pressure and high cholesterol are obesity, alcohol, smoking, a high-fat diet, stress and lack of exercise.

If you reduce your fat calories to 20 to 25 percent of your calorie intake, eat a diet that's mostly whole grains, fresh fruits and vegetables, take a brisk 20-minute walk every day, and cut way down on sugar and refined carbohydrates, I guarantee you'll lose weight. If you make the above diet and lifestyle changes, quit smoking, and keep your alcohol consumption low, it is a near certainty that your blood pressure and cholesterol will drop. If you do all of the above, and your blood pressure and cholesterol are still high, take a good look at the stress in your life, and take steps to reduce it.

CHAPTER 21

Ban Pesticides from Your Life

Chronic exposure to pesticides is a known heart disease risk, but one that most people never think of when they have their lawn doused with chemicals, or spray their garden, go after bugs in the house with a can of spray, or have their house fumigated. If you're pouring poisons down gopher or mole holes, dousing your aphids with pesticides and your dog with flea dip, you're exposing yourself, and your heart, to unacceptable levels of poisons.

These poisons may not kill you on the spot, but they will create free radical damage in your tissues, and accumulate in the body. A study done in the Ukraine of agricultural workers showed that those frequently exposed to pesticides had a higher rate of heart disease as well as a higher rate of abortions and birth defects. There is also evidence that fetal exposure to pesticides can cause congenital heart disease.

OTHER TOXINS PROMOTE HEART DISEASE

Pesticides aren't the only toxins that can cause heart disease. Others, usually found in the workplace, but also in the garage, include solvents, glues and other binding materials, dyes, lacquers, paints, PCBs, metals and vinyl-chloride. In many cases, workers only need to be exposed to fumes or dust from these materials to increase their risk of heart disease.

Please don't take it for granted that, just because you buy a pesticide, herbicide, fungicide, cleaning solvent, paint or other chemical from the hardware store, it's safe. The industries that use these substances are largely unregulated. There are literally thousands of these products on the shelves that have never been tested for safety. In fact, I recommend you assume they are harmful unless you find out otherwise, and avoid contact with skin and avoid breathing the fumes. Even simple household chemicals such as ammonia and chlorine can be harmful.

Another source of chronic exposure to heart-harming substances is air pollution. A number of studies have shown that many thousands of people die each year of heart attacks caused by poor air quality. Granted, their hearts may have been in bad shape to begin with, but a good dose of carbon monoxide can push people over the edge. Try to avoid sitting in traffic and breathing car exhaust, and avoid exercising outside around heavy traffic. Neither your lungs nor your heart will thank you for it!

REDUCE YOUR EXPOSURE

Here are some tips for reducing your exposure to pesticides and other environmental toxins:

- Control fleas on your pets and in your home with substances such as boric acid compounds (now found in most pet stores or call Flea Busters) and aromatic oils such as pennyroyal rather than flea powders.
- If you're a gardener, learn how to do it the organic way. There are plenty of books and magazines on the subject, and local classes are easy to find. You *can* create a beautiful lawn and garden without chemicals, and in the long run you'll have far fewer pest problems.

- Don't drink tap water. (See the chapter on drinking clean water.)
- If you are exposed to pesticides, take a cool shower and drink plenty of clean water to help flush out the poisons.
- Wash, peel or even scrub fruits and vegetables well and eat organic produce whenever possible.
- If you think something at work is making you sick, pursue it. It could be mold or fungus in the heating or cooling system, fumes from wall paneling or carpets, or a co-worker's cigarette smoke.
- Stop using fungicides, herbicides and pesticides. Get out of the habit of blasting indoor and outdoor pests with a can of spray. Learn how to control pests naturally. There's a wealth of information at your library and in your bookstore.
- Don't move in next door to an agricultural field or orchard unless you know it's organic and likely to stay that way.

CHAPTER 22

Do I Need to Say It? Quit Smoking

If you're not convinced that smoking is dangerous to your heart, you haven't read the studies!

SMOKING—THE NUMBER ONE PREVENTABLE RISK

A major scientific review of prevention in health care reform found that cigarette smoking is the major preventable risk factor for cardiovascular disease. Even ignoring this level of human misery, heart disease costs approximately 128 billion dollars every year in treatment and lost productivity.

SMOKING AND FIBRINOGEN LEVELS

At least ten large studies have shown how a high fibrinogen level is a major risk factor for cardiovascular disease, including atherosclerosis (clogged arteries) and thrombosis (stroke). Fibrinogen is a blood clotting agent. It is at least as important as other well-known factors like cholesterol levels. Fibrinogen levels can be used to assess the severity of coronary artery disease and stroke, and the risk of arteries becoming blocked again after surgery. And, you guessed it: smoking increases fibrinogen levels.

SMOKING WORKS AGAINST ANTIOXIDANTS

Studies continue to reveal the ways in which smoking is a threat to your heart. One study of 44 smokers and 44 nonsmokers, aged between 22 and 28, showed that smokers had lower levels of vitamin C than nonsmokers. Furthermore, when smokers took vitamin C there was no corresponding rise in their blood levels of vitamin C. As reported in the *British Journal of Nutrition*, this finding indicates that smoking lowers the body's antioxidant status as well as bombarding it with very high levels of the harmful substances that antioxidants help to neutralize.

LOW TAR STILL MEANS HIGH RISK

Regular or low tar—it makes no difference, your risk of a heart attack is still a hefty four times greater than that of nonsmokers. This was the finding of a study published in the *British Medical Journal*. When it comes to heart disease, the choice is not about tar levels, it's about stopping now!

PASSIVE SMOKING CREATES ACTIVE RISK

An article in the *Journal of the American Medical Association* reviewed the research on passive smoking and heart disease. Predictably, it concluded that nonsmokers exposed to secondhand smoke on a daily basis have an increased risk of heart disease, nonfatal and fatal. The danger lies in the cocktail of chemicals in cigarette smoke, which include carbon monoxide, nicotine, and hydrocarbons. The result of breathing in these noxious chemicals is decreased oxygen supply to the heart and compromised heart function. In addition, secondhand smoke increases blood clotting activity and artery lesions, and promotes tissue damage following heart attacks. Secondhand smoke? You don't want even a whiff of it!

Making Quitting Easier

Did you know your senses of taste and smell improve greatly if you give up smoking? That's just one more incentive to quit. Fortunately, there are several strategies to try, although statistics show the most successful method is actually to go cold turkey.

Other methods include nicotine patches, which can be prescribed by your doctor. These give a gradually reduced dose of nicotine over the course of a few months. This is designed to wean you off the nicotine, which is highly addictive.

It makes sense to support your body while you reduce its dependency. Funnily enough, raw, shelled, unsalted sunflower seeds can help. Keep them with you to munch on whenever you feel a craving for a cigarette. Sunflower seeds are rich in B complex vitamins and zinc. These nutrients help to lower blood acidity and lessen the stress of withdrawal on your body.

It's a good idea to use supplements as an antistress measure while you are quitting smoking. Recommended daily are: 50 mg of B complex; 2,000 mg of vitamin C; 15 mg zinc, taken at night to avoid interference with copper absorption; and 800 mg of magnesium per day, with 400 mg taken just before bedtime to help you relax.

Making the decison to quit smoking is a major move toward a healthier heart and a healthier life in general.

REFERENCES

Abbott, Lisa, et al., "Magnesium Deficiency in Alcoholism: Possible Contribution to Osteoporosis and Cardiovascular Disease in Alcoholics," *Alcoholism: Clinical and Experimental Research,* September/October 1994;18(5):1076–1082.

Baird, I., et al., "The Effects of Ascorbic Acid and Flavonoids on the Occurrence of Symptoms Normally Associated with the Common Cold," *Am. J. Clin. Nutr.,* 1979, 32, pp. 1686–90.

Bellizzi, M., et al., "Vitamin E and Coronary Heart Disease: The European Paradox," *European Journal of Clinical Nutrition,* 1994, 48:822–831.

Bland, J., "The Nutritional Effects of Free Radical Pathology," in 1986—*A Year in Nutritional Medicine,* New Canaan, Conn.: Keats, 1986, p. 304.

Bordia, A., "The Effect of Vitamin C on Blood Lipids, Fibrinolytic Activity and Platelet Adhesiveness in Patients with Coronary Artery Disease," *Atherosclerosis,* 1980, 35:181–187.

Braverman, E., et al., *The Healing Nutrients Within: Facts, Findings, and New Research on Amino Acids,* New Canaan, Conn.: Keats Publishing, 1987, p. 90.

Bulpitt, C., "Vitamin and Blood Pressure," *Journal of Hypertension Theory and Practice,* 1992, A14(1&2):119-38.

Chope, H., et al., "Nutritional Status of the Aging," *American Journal of Public Health,* 1955, 44:61–67.

Elin, R., "Magnesium: The Forgotten Nutrient," *The Nutrition Report,* February 1995;7/"Magnesium: The 5th But Forgotten Electrolyte," *American Journal of Clinical Pathology,* 1994; 102(5):616–622.

Fogarty, M., "Garlic's Potential Role in Reducing Heart Disease," *British Journal of Clinical Practice,* 1993, 47(2):64–65.

Gadkari, J.V., "The Effect of Ingestion of Raw Garlic on Serum Cholesterol Level, Clotting Time and Fibrinolytic Activity in Normal Subjects," *Journal of Postgraduate Medicine,* 1991, 37 (3):128–131.

Gillum, Richard F., "Dental Disease and Coronary Artery Disease," *American Heart Journal,* December 1994;1267.

"Insights into the Pathogenesis and Prevention of Coronary

Artery Disease," O'Keefe, James H., Jr., M.D., et al., Mayo Clinic Proceedings, January 1995;70:69–79.

Jacques, P., "Effects of Vitamin C on HDL and Blood Pressure," Journal of the American College of Nutrition, 1990, 9(5): 554/Abstract 106.

Kanazawa, T., et al., "Anti-atherogenicity of Soybean Protein," Annals of New York Academy of Science 676, 1993:202–214.

Lip, G.Y.H., "Fibrinogen and Cardiovascular Disorders," Quarterly Journal of Medicine, 1995;88:155–165.

Lou, F., et al., "A Study on Tea Pigment in the Prevention of Atherosclerosis," Preventive Medicine, 1992, 21(3):333.

MacRury, S., et al., "Seasonal and Climatic Variation in Cholesterol and Vitamin C: Effect of Vitamin C Supplementation," Scottish Medical Journal, 1992, 37(2):49–52.

Norwell, D.Y., et al., "Garlic, Vampires and CHD," Osteopath. Ann., 1984, 12:276–280.

"Research Offers Evidence of Vitamin E Cardiac Benefit," Medical Tribune, Nov. 21, 1994;8.

Riemersma, R., "Risk of Angina Pectoris and Plasma Concentrations of Vitamins A, C, and E and Carotene," Lancet, 1991: 337(8732):1–5.

Rimm, E., et al., "Vitamin E Consumption and the Risk of Coronary Heart Disease in Men," New England Journal of Medicine, 1993, 328:1450–1456.

Serna, Gaspar De La, M.D., "Fibrinogen: A New Major Risk Factor for Cardiovascular Disease: A Review of the Literature," The Journal of Family Practice, November 1994;39(5): 468–477.

Slavin, J., "Nutritional Benefits of Soy Protein and Soy Fiber," Journal of the American Dietetic Association 91, 1991:816–819.

Stampfer, M., et al., "Vitamin E Consumption and the Risk of Coronary Disease in Women," New England Journal of Medicine, 1993, 328(20):1444–1449.

Steiner, M., et al., "Vitamin E—An Inhibitor of Platelet Release Action," J. Clin. Invest., 1976, 57:732–7.

Van Poppel, Geert, et al., "Antioxidants and Coronary Heart Disease," Annals of Medicine, 1994;26:429–434.

Verschuren, W. M. Monique, MSc., "Serum Total Cholesterol and Long-Term Coronary Heart Disease Mortality in Different Cultures: Twenty-Five-Year Follow-Up of the Seven Countries Study," *JAMA*, July 12, 1995;274(2):131–136.

Wilcox, G., et al., "Oestrogenic Effects of Plant Foods in Post-menopausal Women," *British Medical Journal* 30, 1990: 905–906.

INDEX

Dr. Earl Mindell's

What You Should Know About...
series
in print or forthcoming